Plant-Forward keto

Flexible Recipes + Meal Plans
to **Add Variety, Stay Healthy**
& **Eat the Rainbow**

LIZ MACDOWELL

VICTORY BELT PUBLISHING
Las Vegas

—— • ——

Thank you so much to all my friends and family for your overwhelming love and support. And a special thank you to my husband for all of the taste tests, grocery runs, kitchen cleanups, and pep talks along the way.

—— • ——

First published in 2022 by Victory Belt Publishing Inc.

ISBN-13: 978-1-628601-51-0

Cover design by Justin-Aaron Velasco

Interior design by Kat Lannom and Eli San Juan

Illustrations by Eli San Juan

Meat protein topper recipes on pages 184 to 201 by Launie Kettler

Meat protein topper recipe photos by Tatiana Briceag

Printed in Canada

TC 0122

Table of Contents

———— • ————

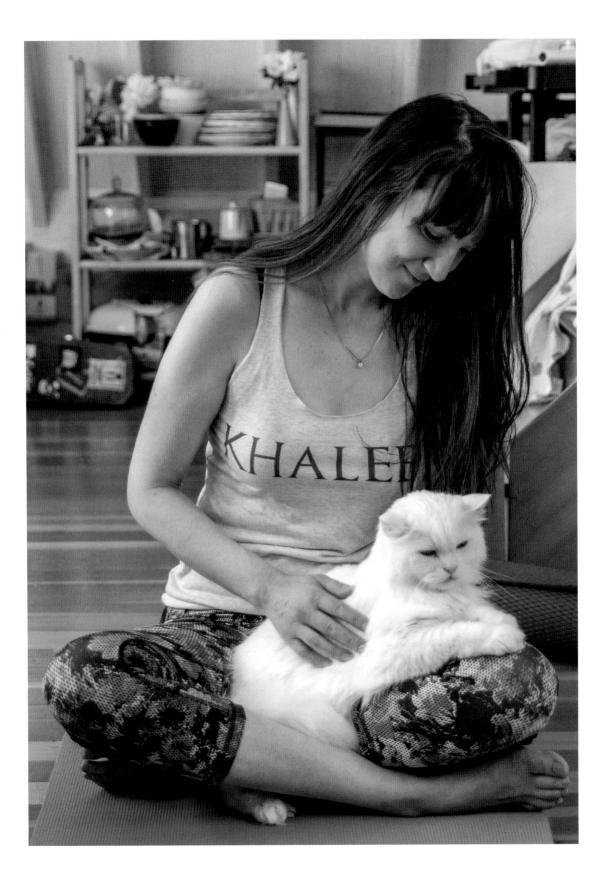

Introduction

——— • ———

Hi, friend! I'm so happy you found this book. If you read my previous book, *Vegan Keto,* or follow me on social media, you may already know a bit about me and how I came to eat a vegan keto diet. If not, hello and welcome; it's nice to meet you! Here's a little bit about why I follow a plant-based ketogenic way of eating.

——— • ———

I first stumbled across ketogenic diets in 2012, after a somewhat disastrous attempt at a high-carb, raw vegan diet that the self-proclaimed "experts" on YouTube assured me would fix all of my health problems. Instead of clear skin, boundless energy, perfect digestion, and rapid weight loss, I experienced constant extreme fatigue, insatiable hunger, the chills, a lot of what I am going to gently refer to as "moodiness," and (much to my dismay) weight *gain*.

As embarrassed as I am to admit it, I often think that if it wasn't for the 10 pounds I gained during that six-week period, I would have kept going despite the other awful side effects. Anyone who has been desperate to fix their health and/or lose weight can probably relate to that feeling. Thankfully, the weight gain forced me to re-evaluate how my current diet was impacting my well-being, and I started looking for alternatives.

Because I tend to exist in extremes, my natural response to a high-carb diet failure was to look into low-carb diets. I had played around with Atkins (also plant-based, which meant my meals consisted of a lot of peanut butter, cheese, and eggs and not much else) in the late 1990s and experienced moderate success, so that diet became my launching-off point. A few internet rabbit holes later and I discovered keto.

At the risk of sounding overly dramatic, keto changed my life. I lost the extra weight that plagued me, the pain and swelling in my joints vanished, I felt more clear-headed than ever, and I finally understood what people meant when they said they were "regular." If you also have IBS, you'll likely relate there. I also experienced a balancing of my once-volatile blood sugar levels and a bunch of other smaller effects that are too boring to list here. Keto really helped me understand what it is like to feel (I assume) "normal." So, despite it being a little out-there, I stuck with a plant-based, very-low-carb way of eating.

I'm not sharing this story to talk about how great keto is and how terrible high-carb vegan diets are. In fact, many studies show that high-carb vegan diets can be incredibly beneficial for improving blood sugar control, metabolic markers, and cardiovascular health—the very same improvements people notice on ketogenic diets! Clearly, high-carb plant-based diets have their place in the nutrition world. I just happen to be one of the people for whom a high-carb diet is not the right approach.

In this same vein, I don't think ketogenic diets are right for everyone. I know people who never felt well while in ketosis despite "doing everything right." Some of them started to notice benefits when they increased their carbohydrate intake to the point of eating a low-carb, but not ketogenic, diet. Others started thriving when they took a more medium-carb approach. The point is, we are all different, and it's impossible to know what will work for your body without doing a little experimentation.

My own experience with trying to dial in what works best for me has taken many different forms. While I currently eat a predominantly keto-friendly and entirely plant-based diet, there are days when my body seems to function better with some additional carbohydrates. (More on that later!) I have also increased my baseline intake of carbs over the years as my fitness goals and lifestyle have changed.

While my first book reflected where I was when I started keto (pretty strict with my net carbs, with little wiggle room and a lot of tracking), the recipes in this book mirror the way I eat today—increased flexibility in meals with a larger variety of vegetables and modifications to adjust the carbohydrate content.

This book also recognizes that while many of us follow a completely plant-based diet, not everyone does. Many people live in mixed-diet households where many accommodations must be made at mealtime for different ways of eating. Many more incorporate some form of animal product in at least one meal per day. With this in mind, this book contains suggestions for using a broader variety of proteins for those who eat eggs or dairy, and even a section of animal protein recipes developed by a super talented recipe developer. So, if you happen to be plant-based but your spouse and kids are not, you can make one entrée and two proteins instead of two completely different entrées.

However, if you eat a totally plant-based diet, you can still make every single main recipe in this book. I just want everyone to feel as good as possible!

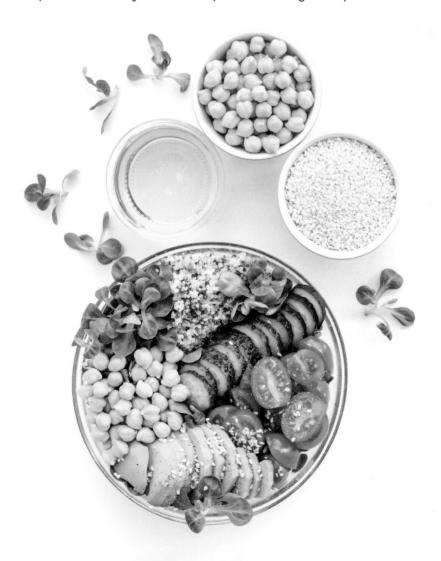

What Does Plant-Forward Mean?

You may have seen the hashtag #plantforward floating around on social media and wondered how it's different from #plantpowered or #plantbased. Or maybe the title of this book was your introduction to this phrase! Either way, I thought I'd take a moment to explain what plant-forward means to me (outside of the hashtag) and why it's in the title of this book.

The basic idea is that *plant-forward* describes a way of eating that puts plants on your plate first. It sounds super simple, and that's because it is. Unlike the qualifiers *plant-based* and *plant-strong,* both of which imply some level of vegetarianism, there is no dogma or lifestyle proclamation attached to *plant-forward.* You can be a vegan and plant-forward, or be an omnivore and plant-forward. The gates are open, and everyone is welcome to come on in and add more plant foods to their diets.

Plant-forward *keto* takes this idea of building meals around plant foods and extends it to a ketogenic diet. So, the plants featured in these recipes are all relatively low in carbohydrates and sugar. Plant-forward keto also embraces the more flexible side of ketogenic diets, recognizing that we all have different macronutrient needs: some of us are happy at the lower end of the carb spectrum, while others thrive when eating closer to their upper carb limit. In this vein, you'll note many meal options contain higher-carb vegetable and fruit substitutions to accommodate all types of keto dieters, as well as those looking for general low(er)-carb meals.

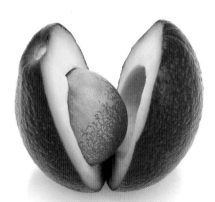

Who Is Plant-Forward Keto For?

Truly, it's for pretty much everyone. This book isn't just for vegans or vegetarians. Whether you are completely plant-based, cutting back on meat, or just trying to add more vegetables to your regular keto meals, plant-forward keto can be right for you!

Keto Basics

While you probably already know something about ketogenic diets, I figure it's worth covering the basics. In short, a ketogenic diet is a high-fat and low-carbohydrate way of eating that shifts your body from burning carbohydrates as its primary source of fuel to a state in which it preferentially burns fats in a process called *nutritional ketosis.* Restricting your intake of carbohydrates and forcing your body to burn fats for fuel drastically decreases the amount of insulin required to regulate your blood sugar levels.

Because of its insulin-stabilizing effects, many people find that a state of nutritional ketosis is beneficial for weight loss, decreasing inflammation,[2] stabilizing hormone levels,[3] and even regulating mood.[4]

While you *can* make a ketogenic diet as complicated as you want with supplements and feeding schedules and exact macronutrient targets, at its core keto is pretty simple. The basic principles are these: eat lots of fat, a moderate amount of protein, and few enough carbs that you stay in ketosis. That's it. There are no supplements you *have* to take to get/stay in ketosis, no exact macronutrient ratios you *have* to stick to, and no list of foods you absolutely *have* to avoid.

That being said, there are plenty of keto guidelines out there; I'll go over them quickly so you have a starting point in case this is your first foray into ketogenic diets. But let's start with how plant-forward keto differs from regular keto.

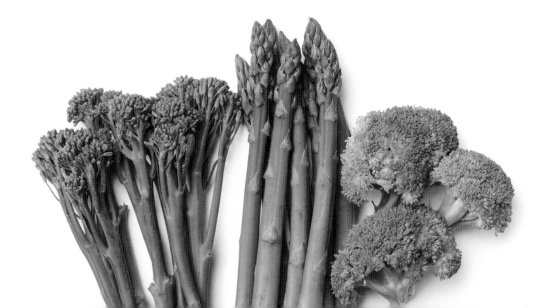

How Plant-Forward Keto Differs from Classic Keto

A classic ketogenic diet tends to focus mostly on keeping carb intake very low and fat intake very high. The focus is less on the types of foods eaten and more on the macros. As a result, many traditional keto diets tend to load up on meat, cheese, and eggs (because those foods contain little to no carbohydrates), with vegetables and other plant foods as more of an afterthought. Plant-forward keto, as the name suggests, places greater focus on eating whole plant foods with less emphasis on macros and less attention to minimizing carbs.

Those of you eating a plant-based ketogenic diet are likely already following a form of plant-forward keto (unless you are literally just eating protein powder and oil…which I have seen on more than one social media feed), but plant-forward keto doesn't mean you cannot eat animal products. However, animal products would be considered more of a topping or a side instead of the main component of the meal.

There are no specific rules to eating a plant-based keto diet. The general idea is that plant foods simply take up more space on your plate than anything else and form the foundation for your meals instead of only appearing as an occasional side. This means that while you will still be in a state of nutritional ketosis on plant-forward keto, you may find yourself increasing your carbohydrate intake a bit in order to incorporate more whole plant foods.

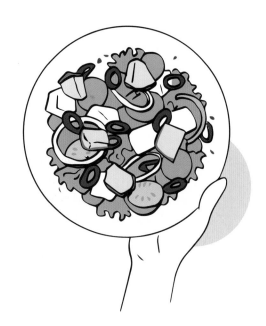

Wait, *More* Carbs on Keto?

Misconceptions I see quite often in the ketosphere are that carbs are inherently bad and need to be avoided at all costs, and that you cannot consume anything with any amount of sugar if you want to stay in ketosis. Carbohydrates are natural components of the foods we eat. Broccoli contains sugar, spinach contains sugar, cheese contains sugar...and even eggs contain sugar (about half a gram each)! Unless you are eating only unseasoned meat and oil and drinking nothing but water, you are going to be consuming some form of sugar, and that's not a bad thing.

There are plenty of reasons to eat toward your upper carb limit on a ketogenic diet. First, it's much easier, especially if you are vegetarian or vegan. Unless you are drinking straight oil (which some people do—whatever floats your boat), pretty much every vegetarian or vegan food contains carbs. So, breaking free of the 20-gram limit can make following a keto diet drastically easier for plant-based eaters. That's not to say it's impossible otherwise; it's just keto on hard mode.

If the idea of eating more carbohydrates is a little stressful to you, I get it. Years of reading about the evils of sugar and carbohydrates definitely makes me stop and think every time I am about to add some berries to a smoothie or beans to a stew. It's the exact response I had to consuming so much fat when I first started eating a ketogenic diet after living through the fat-phobic 1990s. When so much attention is given to macronutrients, we tend to forget what they actually are— sources of nutrition.

It's easy to demonize carbohydrates and sugar and thus want to categorically avoid them, but to me, this is not a helpful way to think. For one, foods are not inherently "bad" or "good," and setting up a paradigm of food having some kind of morality doesn't do anyone any favors. Secondly, carbohydrates are a core component of vegetables, fruits, beans, nuts, and seeds, which are all incredibly nutrient-dense. Categorically eschewing carbohydrates eliminates a lot of really beneficial (and delicious) foods.

Instead of trying to minimize carbohydrate intake, I like to think in terms of getting the most nutritional bang for my carbohydrate buck. So, while I really love eating grapes and apples, they're both pretty high in carbohydrates, and "spending" my carbohydrate allowance on foods like these won't provide as much nutritional benefit as choosing jicama, cucumber, celery, or carrots as a snack instead.

Keto by the Numbers

Often, when we think of ketogenic diets, we think of that 20-gram net carb target that has become so ubiquitous. Twenty grams started out as the goal for the induction phase of many low-carb diets, and it's a number at which most people can easily achieve ketosis. So, it's easy to think that ketosis starts and ends here.

In truth, most people can enter into (and maintain) nutritional ketosis by eating between 20 and 50 grams of net carbohydrates per day. Those who exercise with any regularity are usually able to consume higher amounts of carbohydrates and still maintain ketosis, often exceeding this 50-gram threshold. On hikes through the White Mountains of New Hampshire, I've managed to stay in a light state of ketosis while eating up to 75 grams of net carbs in a day, though this is far from a regular occurrence.

When you're starting out on a ketogenic diet, the closer you stay to the 20-gram mark (or lower), the quicker you will enter nutritional ketosis, so many people begin with a daily number of 20 to 30 grams. In time, this range can prove a little too restrictive for those who want to incorporate more plant foods into their diet or be able to enjoy a little more variety in their snacks. To make a ketogenic way of eating a bit more sustainable long term, I like to suggest eating around 20 to 30 grams per day in the beginning and then finding out what your carb tolerance is and eating closer to that number once you've become fat-adapted.

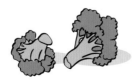

Is There Magic in 20 Grams of Net Carbs?

I want to make it clear that there is nothing magical about the number 20. If you eat 21 grams of carbs in a day, you are not going to be arrested by the Keto Police and thrown in Keto Jail. You can certainly make 20 grams of carbs (net or otherwise) your goal, but don't feel bad if that amount is a little too low for you, or if that's your goal and you exceed it one day!

On the other hand, I know a few people who like to push the limit and try to consume between 10 and 15 grams of total carbs per day for the first month of returning to ketosis... on a vegan diet! It's pretty hard-core and definitely not the easiest way to do it, but it's speedy and gets the job done. Because we are all so different and thrive on various ways of eating, I think it's worth sharing the many ways to get into ketosis.

Finding Your Carb Tolerance

Your carb tolerance is the upper limit of your net carb consumption where you will still be in ketosis. It's useful to know this number if you want to start incorporating slightly higher-carb foods into your eating plan, or if you just want a little less stress when eating at a restaurant, where sugar can sneak its way onto your plate in loads of ways.

You can find your carb tolerance pretty easily by doing a little self-experimentation. Just increase your daily net carb intake by around 5 grams every few days and test your ketone levels to see at what point you stop producing ketones. The amount of carbs you eat before you no longer stay in ketosis is your upper limit. This threshold will vary based on exercise, so keep that in mind!

The most common ways to test ketone levels are by using ketone sticks/strips or a ketone meter. Ketone sticks are those little plastic strips with a pad at the end that you pee on to determine how many ketones are floating around in your system. A ketone meter is similar to the blood glucose meters people with diabetes use to test their blood sugar levels (and they are often one and the same, but use two different types of test strips). Ketone sticks are definitely the cheaper option, but a ketone meter is far more accurate, especially if you're looking to see how a specific food impacts your ketone production in a narrow window of time. However, the meters and test strips that accompany them are expensive and require you to prick your finger to draw a bit of blood. So, both methods have their pros and cons.

You can also find your carb tolerance without using ketone meters or test strips. Once you've been in ketosis for a long enough period (usually four to eight weeks), you'll be pretty used to how ketosis feels and be able to tell when you are kicked out. I can always tell when I've been kicked out by the way my joints (especially in my hands and knees) swell a bit and become stiff and how my head feels a little clouded—but you may have different telltale signs.

For all of these methods, it's helpful to keep track of what you eat each day as well as how you feel after each meal (and the next morning, which is usually when I start to feel icky).

It's important to note that everyone is unique. Our bodies metabolize carbs differently, so while some people may be able to eat closer to 50 grams of net carbs per day and stay in ketosis, others may have to stick closer to that 20-gram mark. This is especially true of those with extreme metabolic damage or insulin resistance. However, your carb tolerance can change over time. Studies have indicated that following a very-low-carb ketogenic diet can improve insulin resistance and other components of metabolic syndrome.[5]

What's a Net Carb?

The term *net carb(s),* which is short for "net effective carbohydrate(s)," refers to the total number of grams of carbohydrates in foods that impact your blood sugar in a significant way. This is the number most people are talking about when they mention the number of carbs they eat in a day.

In the United States and Canada, this number is calculated by subtracting the grams of fiber and sugar alcohols on a food label from the total number of carbohydrates.

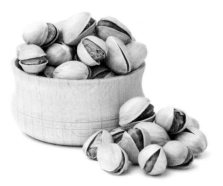

Why I Started Eating More Carbs

If it seems like I'm mentioning eating more carbs a lot here, it's because I want everyone to know that you don't have to be confined to eating just 20 grams per day. When I started out on a plant-based ketogenic diet, I was obsessed with this number. Everything I read on the internet back then said that you had to stay under 20 grams or it wasn't keto. Being totally new to ketogenic diets, I believed this, and I was miserable some days because of it. I would stress out every time I consumed more than that number, and I limited the variety of foods I ate in order to stay within the limit.

Once I increased my intake to around 35 grams, it was like a whole new world opened up at mealtime. I still experienced all of the positive effects of ketosis, but I didn't feel stressed every time I ate something with more carbs—like pistachios instead of super low-carb (but not super wallet-friendly) macadamia nuts—and I didn't have to limit my consumption of vegetables in order to hit that low target.

How Many Calories/Net Carbs/Grams of Protein Should I Eat?

It might seem strange that I've grouped calories, carbohydrates, and protein together, because they are completely different, but the answer for all three is the same: you should eat however many you need. I know: annoying, right? Unfortunately for those of us looking for the easy way to do something, there's no one right answer to these questions. This is because we all have different bodies, genetic makeups, lifestyles, and goals; we also have different caloric and macronutrient needs.

I usually recommend finding a baseline using a macronutrient calculator. These calculators typically take into account your height, weight, age, general body composition, and lifestyle to come up with the approximate number of calories you burn just to keep your body running at its baseline (called your basal metabolic rate, or BMR for short) and the total number of calories you burn in a day with all your activity taken into account (your total daily energy expenditure, or TDEE). They're not perfect by any means, but they give you a good place to start. There are many available online, including one on my blog here: meatfreeketo.com/vegan-keto-macro-calculator.

Once you have this starting point, you can play around with the numbers depending on how you feel. It may take you a while to find the caloric intake and macronutrient ratios that work best for you, but knowing these numbers will make your life easier in the long run. Over time, as you lose weight, gain muscle, and/or change your fitness routine, you may find that you need to go back and readjust your macronutrient and caloric targets.

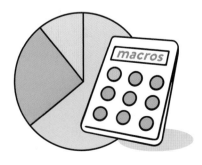

If It's Not Broken, Don't Fix It

I've talked a lot about higher carb targets and carb cycling (and I'll talk even more about that later in this book), but I want to mention here that you absolutely do not have to eat a higher-carb ketogenic diet if you don't want to or if it doesn't feel right to your body. It's totally possible to consume a plant-forward keto diet within the normal 20- to 50-gram net carb range, or even below 20 grams (although it starts to get challenging there).

Many people happily practice a straightforward ketogenic diet without high-carb days for months at a time, taking a break only for a birthday or holiday (if at all!). If you fall into this group, there's no pressure to change things up. Additionally, if you're new to ketogenic diets or pretty far from your weight-loss goal, you may not want to start a carb cycling routine just yet or venture beyond a relatively low target.

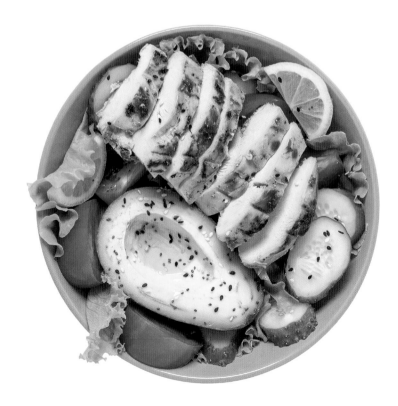

Keto, in All Its Forms

As you may have gathered from social media, there are many ways to get and stay in ketosis, and in this section I'm going to talk about a few of the most common ones. Several of these styles can be combined, so you can do OMAD (one meal a day) and whole-food keto, or combine relaxed keto with intermittent fasting.

You don't have to label the type of ketogenic diet you follow, but it can help to familiarize yourself with these terms, especially when browsing message boards and social media posts.

If It Fits Your Macros (IIFYM)

This way of eating is how I got my start on keto. The idea is that you find your ideal macronutrient ratio, or just your net carb goal, and then eat whatever foods you want to help you achieve this goal. As you may have guessed, this style of eating requires you to track your foods in order to hit those macronutrient targets; however, that's the only real requirement.

The types of foods you eat on IIFYM don't really matter; you could eat entirely whole foods, or entirely packaged convenience foods, or some happy medium between the two. Many people who eat a ketogenic diet do so with the IIFYM mindset.

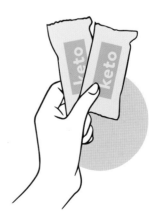

Dirty Keto

Dirty keto basically refers to eating lots of processed foods like protein bars and keto snacks to achieve ketosis. In this style of eating, you may or may not be attached to a certain set of macronutrients, or you may just eat to stay in ketosis.

Dirty keto isn't my favorite term, but it's commonly used and therefore worth mentioning. The reason I don't love saying something is dirty is that it starts to tiptoe along that line of judging food choices. *Dirty* is a word that we subconsciously associate with being bad, and I just don't feel we need to qualify foods in that way. But this is the prevalent term for this way of eating, so here we are.

Clean Keto & Whole-Food Keto

Both of these terms can be used to describe a keto diet that relies on unprocessed whole foods like vegetables, fruits, nuts, some legumes, and maybe animal products. Some people include cold-pressed oils in this way of eating, while others do not.

Typically, a food is considered processed if it cannot be easily re-created in a home kitchen. So, nut butters and nondairy milks would be considered whole foods by this definition, as they can easily be made at home with a blender or food processor. Another way to think about whole foods is that they contain just one ingredient (excluding salt and water), so tofu, tempeh, canned coconut milk, kelp noodles, cheese, nutritional yeast, and psyllium husks are often included in this category as well.

This style of eating also does not require you to stick to a certain set of macronutrients, though you certainly can follow one if you'd like.

You probably saw this coming, but for the same reason I don't love the term *dirty keto,* I feel a little weird saying *clean keto.* I think the name *whole-food keto* gets the same message across without any unnecessary holier-than-thou connotations.

The recipes in this book mostly fall into the category of whole-food keto. This is how I eat most of the time because it's what feels best for my body. That being said, I also follow the 80/20 principle, where around 80 percent of my food intake is whole foods and the remaining 20 percent is comprised of things like mock meats, protein bars, protein powder, and keto treats.

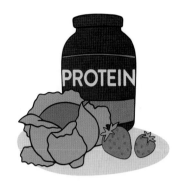

Relaxed Keto

Relaxed keto is my favorite style, and it works really well with a plant-forward low-carb or medium-carb way of eating. It's basically an intuitive way of approaching ketogenic/low-carb/medium-carb diets, where instead of counting calories and grams of carbs, you just eat until you reach satiety, focusing on low-carb foods. So no tracking (or minimal tracking), no stressing, and no scheduling. You eat when you want and however much you need to feel full.

I used to refer to this style as *lazy keto*, but I prefer the more positive association of saying something is *relaxed* as opposed to *lazy*. This is the approach I tend to take most days, though I'll track every so often to see where I am.

Intuitive Eating on Keto

When I work with long-term clients, the goal is usually to transition them to some form of intuitive eating in the long run. It's how animals in the wild eat, it's how our hunter-gatherer ancestors ate, and it's the least stressful way of eating that I've found. It's also one of the most difficult things to adapt to for a lot of us, especially those who tend to eat emotionally and/or have a damaged relationship with eating and food.

The idea of intuitive eating is really basic: eat whatever you want, whenever you want, in whatever quantities you want. Of course, this is much easier said than done and is something that can take years to learn, especially in a culture where we are bombarded by hyperpalatable foods that are designed to override our bodies' hunger cues so that no matter how full we are, we are always hungry for more.

It may seem contradictory to talk about intuitive eating in the same breath as ketogenic diets, since in order to enter into nutritional ketosis, you have to at least somewhat limit the foods you eat, but I think keto can provide a nice framework for learning how to eat intuitively. One reason ketogenic diets can be so beneficial is the main side effect that so many people report: a reduction or elimination of cravings. For me, after more than a decade of trying endless diets, keto was the only thing that eliminated my cravings for carb-laden foods and helped me stop the cycle of emotional eating and bingeing. Keto opened the door for me to start eating more intuitively and less emotionally.

A way to practice intuitive eating on a ketogenic diet is to adopt a relaxed approach and stop tracking or counting, focusing predominantly on eating what your body craves from the list of low-carb foods. Don't worry about hitting your macro ratio perfectly or not going over your calories for the day; just focus on eating low-carb foods. You can take this approach from the start, but you may not actually get into ketosis, so I find it's best to start working toward intuitive eating once you've been on a ketogenic diet for at least a month.

If abandoning tracking completely is a little too much for you to start, you could dip your toes into intuitive eating by focusing on keeping track of net carbs. Still try to eat the low-carb foods you want at the times you want (no need to worry about intermittent fasting here!), but be mindful of your net carb intake. After you've become comfortable eating this way, try letting go of tracking net carbs as well.

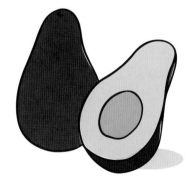

Scheduled Eating on Keto

In addition to a number of styles of eating, there are a few types of eating schedules that people often follow. You don't have to follow any of these to eat a ketogenic diet, but they're worth mentioning.

Intermittent Fasting

Intermittent fasting (IF) isn't limited to those on ketogenic diets, but many people who are on keto utilize IF as a health and fitness tool. Basically, intermittent fasting is a fancy way of saying "eating within a certain window of time." You can make it more complicated if you like, but at its core, it's just timing when you eat. People typically practice intermittent fasting to promote fat-burning and weight loss, reduce inflammation, and control appetite and hunger cues by regulating the hormone leptin (among other things).

The most common form of IF is to fast for 16 hours and eat in an 8-hour window, typically represented as 16:8. You may be practicing some form of intermittent fasting without even realizing it! If you tend not to eat breakfast and aren't a big night eater, then you might already be eating within an 8-hour window.

I often eat in a 16:8 window because I'm just not big on eating in the morning (it just doesn't feel right to my body), but I also find that being too rigid with my eating windows usually causes more stress than it's worth, so I'm not strict about timing my meals.

IF Is Not for Everyone

While intermittent fasting is a helpful tool for many people, it can be problematic for others. People with two X-chromosomes and a case of estrogen dominance may find that fasting leaves them feeling tired and hangry. So, if you try IF and it just doesn't seem to work for you, it's likely that it isn't a good match. I know folks online have a tendency to tell you that you're doing something "wrong" if IF isn't working for you, but not every way of eating works for every individual!

Alternate-Day Fasting

Another somewhat aggressive form of intermittent fasting is alternate-day fasting, where you eat every other day. Some people consume broth and tea or coffee (with creamer if they want) on their fasting day, while others only drink water.

One Meal a Day

Like intermittent fasting, one meal a day (OMAD) isn't limited to ketogenic diets, but there is a lot of overlap between those who practice OMAD and those on ketogenic or low-carb diets. OMAD is a subset of IF whereby all of the day's food is consumed within one meal. It's basically the hard-core version of IF. It follows the same basic idea of eating all of your food within a small window, but instead of a 16:8 window, it's a 22:2 or 23:1 window.

Many people use OMAD for weight loss, as eating all of their food for the day at once makes it feel like a feast, so it's easier to keep calories lower. Eating in such a small window also allows the body to direct the energy it would normally spend digesting meals to regenerating cells.

Intermittent fasting and fasting in general are interesting topics. If you want to learn more about them or give fasting a try, I highly recommend *The Complete Guide to Fasting,* by Dr. Jason Fung.

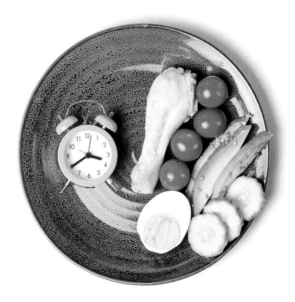

Carb Cycling

As I mentioned before, I like to think of keto as a tool that I can use to help me achieve my health and fitness goals. Another tool that I've found to be incredibly helpful is carb cycling, which is a great way to make ketogenic diets more sustainable, especially for those who are active.

As with ketogenic diets in general, carb cycling can be as simple or as complicated as you want. Because I get more questions about carb cycling than any other aspect of keto, I'm going to devote more time to it than the other keto variations, but focus on the simpler implementations of this practice that will be beneficial to a wide range of people.

What Is Carb Cycling?

As you may have inferred from the name, *carb cycling* refers to alternating between a set amount of lower-carb (or keto) days and higher-carb days. While you can certainly practice carb cycling outside the bounds of a ketogenic diet, I'm going to focus on how this practice can be used in conjunction with keto.

Carb cycling on a ketogenic diet is often referred to as a cyclical ketogenic diet (CKD). The easiest way to practice cyclical keto is by choosing one day a week to be your high-carb day and then eating your typical ketogenic diet the rest of the week. For many people, this is a weekend day, but you can pick any day that makes sense for you.

If you work out a lot, you may want to have more than one higher-carb day in a week, matching your workout schedule. I know some people who make each heavy workout day a higher-carb day, while moderate workout days might be moderate-carb days and rest days are very low-carb. You can experiment over time to optimize carb cycling for your lifestyle.

The bottom line is that there isn't one correct way to practice carb cycling in conjunction with ketosis. It depends entirely on your particular metabolism, lifestyle, activity level, and fitness goals. I want to make this point clear because I see so many websites talking about carb cycling as if there's only one correct way to do it, and that's simply not true.

Why Carb Cycle?

There are a few main reasons someone might start adding higher-carb days to an otherwise low-carb or ketogenic eating plan. The first is to reduce cravings for higher-carb foods. I think this is the most obvious benefit. If you have a scheduled day when you plan on having some french fries or pasta, you're less likely to indulge in those foods during the rest of the week.

The second most common reason most people start a CKD is to support their workouts and fitness goals. The idea is to replenish liver glycogen stores that are depleted through your workouts on the high-carb day.

Another rationale for considering carb cycling, especially if you've been on a ketogenic protocol for a while, is that some studies have indicated it can prevent the dip in metabolism that can occur in long-term low-carb dieters. This effect is enhanced by overfeeding carbohydrates.[7]

So, eating over your daily caloric expenditure on your high-carb day can actually help with long-term weight loss. This is also the reason many people find that a cheat day or high-carb day can help them break through a weight-loss plateau.

Finally, some people, particularly those who menstruate, those with certain hormone imbalances, and those with thyroid imbalances, may find that they feel tired, irritable, and somewhat lethargic on long-term very-low-carb diets. Introducing higher-carb days can alleviate some of that fatigue and discomfort.

Won't Carb Cycling Kick Me Out of Ketosis?

Most likely, yes—but that's okay! You do not need to be in ketosis 100 percent of the time to glean benefits from this way of eating. Additionally, you can typically get back into ketosis within a day or two. If you find that you are unable to easily transition back into ketosis after a high-carb day, moving to a cycle where you have a high-carb day every two weeks may work better for you.

As mentioned previously, being knocked out of ketosis every once in a while can actually help preserve your metabolic rate and aid in long-term weight loss.

How to Get Started on Carb Cycling

If you're brand-new to keto or low/moderate-carb diets, I wouldn't recommend carb cycling right away. Usually, it takes about a month to become fat-adapted, where your body has fully adjusted to its new low-carb existence. At this point, re-entering a state of nutritional ketosis will be much easier than it was during the adaptation period. Additionally, the first month is the time in any new dietary protocol where cravings hit the hardest and can easily derail your progress.

Once you've made it past the first month on a ketogenic diet, starting to carb cycle is really easy: just pick a day and eat more carbs. Like I mentioned before, cyclical ketogenic diets are only as complicated as you want to make them, so there's nothing wrong with just eating a bunch of carbs one day and seeing how it goes. If you want to track calories and macros on that day, you can definitely do so, but it's not necessary.

What Kinds of Foods Should I Eat on a High-Carb Day?

This is really up to you; you can play around to see what feels best. I like to eat in the same plant-forward way but incorporate more beans, fruit, and starches into my meals. So, I might add chickpeas to a stew, or substitute sweet potato for butternut squash, or make sweet potato fries in my air fryer. I also use these days to enjoy some of the higher-carb keto treats that are available nowadays. From cereals to sandwich cookies to ice cream, there are so many commercially available sugar-free products that can easily be incorporated into a higher-carb day without totally blowing up my blood sugar.

On the other hand, you may want to use this day as an opportunity to indulge in some traditional comfort treats with real sugar that you may be missing. I say it with pretty much everything, but it really is all about what feels best for you and your body and what will help you achieve your goals.

How High Is "High-Carb"?

Buckle up, because this is going to be another annoyingly vague answer: it depends. Most of my high-carb days are around 75 to 150 grams of net carbs (depending on how much exercise I do), and that seems to be the sweet spot for me. Anything higher than that and I start to feel sick, which is the exact opposite of how I want to feel.

For you, this number is likely going to be different. If you are intensely sensitive to carbs, you might want to start at 50 to 75 grams of net carbs on a high-carb day. If you are using your high-carb day(s) to lift lots of heavy weights, you may want to start at 200 grams. It really depends on your particular metabolism, lifestyle, and fitness goals. Like carb tolerance, caloric intake, and macronutrient targets, this is one of those things that you'll have to play around with to see what works best for you.

If you are trying to stay within a caloric target, keep in mind that you will want to reduce your fat intake on high-carb days to make up for the additional calories from the extra carbs you are eating. This doesn't mean you should avoid fats altogether, but you don't need to add extra oil to a stir-fry or extra coconut cream to a smoothie in order to hit a fat target.

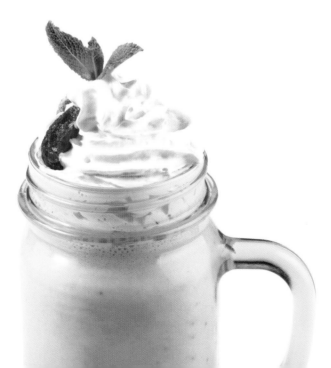

Sample Carb Cycling Schedules

Here are a few examples of how you could schedule carb cycling in the context of a ketogenic or low-carb diet. These are just general guidelines for matching your carb intake to your lifestyle and workout intensity, and you should modify them to fit your lifestyle and workout schedule based on how you feel.

Basic 6 Days Keto, 1 Day High-Carb

- Monday–Saturday: 25–50g net carbs
- Sunday: 100–150g net carbs

Simple Cyclical Ketogenic Diet for Working Out

- Monday (heavy lifting): 200g net carbs
- Tuesday (rest day): 25–50g net carbs
- Wednesday (cardio): 75g net carbs
- Thursday (light yoga): 25–50g net carbs
- Friday (light cardio): 25–50g net carbs
- Saturday (cardio): 75g net carbs
- Sunday (rest day): 25–50g net carbs

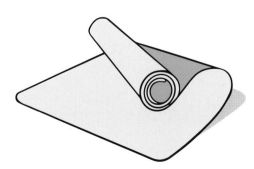

A Note on Working Out on Keto

If you have been doing keto for a while and are totally fat-adapted, then you can skip this box—this message isn't for you. However, if you are new to ketogenic diets or are getting back into nutritional ketosis after some time off, you may want to go easy on the exercise for the first few weeks. That doesn't mean you can't work out at all, just that you might want to keep your workouts at a moderate level.

It can take a few weeks to a couple of months to become fully fat-adapted, and during this time your body may struggle during exercise. However, studies show that ketogenic diets can actually improve performance for fat-adapted endurance athletes, especially during training periods of high-volume, low-to-moderate-intensity workouts.[8]

While low-carb diets can benefit endurance athletes in the long run, athletes who participate primarily in strength-based exercise may find that a super low-carbohydrate diet hinders their performance, as heavy lifting is a glycogen-demanding activity. Additionally, as insulin is beneficial for building muscle, those looking to add muscle mass may find that staying in ketosis all the time makes hypertrophy (building muscle) too much of a challenge. These types of athletes are prime candidates for a carb cycling routine that is tailored to their workout schedule.

Sustaining or Transitioning off Keto

Making Keto Sustainable for You

One of the most common questions that pops up in my inbox is, "How do you eat a ketogenic diet long term without getting bored?" The simplest answer is that you have to find what works best for you individually. After the first month or two, after your body has become fat-adapted, if you find that the way you are practicing keto is getting boring or making you long for change—despite feeling good for your body—then it might be time to make an adjustment!

For some people, this might look like ditching the meal plans and macro counts and focusing on eating keto-friendly foods. For others, it could be scheduling a high-carb day every week or two to deal with cravings in a controlled way. Whichever style of eating a ketogenic diet feels best to you is the way that will be the most sustainable.

For me, 20 grams of net carbs per day just wasn't sustainable, not even in the first few months. It was too low for me to have consistent energy for working out and to be able to eat the variety of vegetables and fruits that felt good to me. So, a couple of months after starting keto, I increased my daily net carb intake to 35 grams per day. As my activity level increased, I played around with carb cycling and increasing my net carbs so I could be as active as I wanted. I also started eating more intuitively and mindfully, stopped tracking for long periods of time, and just went by how my body felt. When I'm not as active, or when I'm trying to reduce inflammation after a day (or a week during the holidays) of indulging, I'll lower my net carbs and start tracking for a bit. It's about finding the balance that works for you.

There are also individuals for whom sticking with a more classic style of keto (without high-carb days or an increase in overall carbs) works best, and that's great, too! I've said it before, and I'll say it again: the most sustainable way of eating is the one that feels best for your body.

Is Keto Forever?

For some people, especially those with an autoimmune disease or other chronic condition, a ketogenic way of eating may be a lifelong commitment. If you fall into one of these categories, how long to continue keto is something you should discuss with your primary care physician or medical team.

Otherwise, keto can be a great tool to help you achieve your weight-loss goals, regulate hunger cues, and balance your relationship with food and eating, but you may find that it's not a totally sustainable long-term solution for you. So what happens when you've reached your goals and you want to transition off keto but don't want to slide back into the high-carb way of eating that came before?

Like most topics in the realm of nutrition, there isn't one right answer here. When transitioning away from a ketogenic diet, you can take an endless number of paths, but I'm going to talk about just two of them here: low-carb and medium-carb ways of eating.

You may notice that I don't mention going back to your previous way of eating. I'm going to say right out of the gate that I don't recommend this path for the majority of people. For most of us, our previous diets were what led us to feel terrible enough to want to try keto. However, if you happen to be in the minority of people who tried keto just to see what it was like and were thriving on your previous way of eating, then you should be able to transition back without any issues.

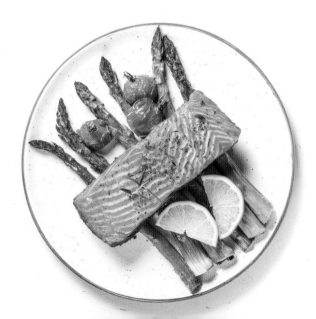

How to Transition off Keto

It may seem odd that a keto cookbook would dedicate an entire section to how to stop eating a ketogenic diet, but I think it's a really important topic. Most people who try keto and get great results might not want to stay on a fully keto plan for the rest of their lives. So how does it work?

In a nutshell, transitioning off keto is as simple as eating more carbohydrates. That's it. That's all you need to do to permanently kick yourself out of ketosis: just eat more carbs, and then keep eating more carbs.

Don't worry—I'm not just going to leave it there. In my experience of working with nutrition clients over nearly ten years, I've found that the best way to transition off a ketogenic diet is slowly, over the course of two to four weeks. Yes, you can just start eating a bunch of carbs one day, but I've noticed that the people who jump right back into a higher-carb way of eating tend to find themselves right back in old eating patterns quickly. And with these old eating patterns comes weight gain and the negative side effects that accompany it. Giving yourself a few weeks to change up your way of eating allows enough time to establish new habits and work toward that ultimate goal of intuitive eating. Another benefit to easing carbs back into your meals is that you can find that sweet spot of carb intake where you don't experience cravings or carb binges.

For those who eventually want to transition from keto to a low-carb or medium-carb way of eating, I've included some medium-carb plant foods in this book, both in the food lists and in suggestions in some of the recipes.

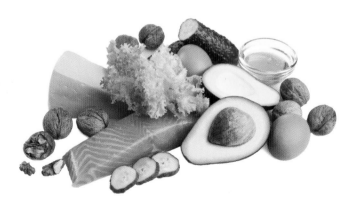

Transitioning to a Low-Carb Diet

Low-carb diets that don't bring you all the way to nutritional ketosis have been trending on and off for a while now, and for good reason. Lower-carb diets have demonstrated many of the same reported benefits of ketogenic diets, like reduced appetite,[9] improved cholesterol and triglyceride levels,[10] and improved blood sugar control.[11] The benefits that general low-carb ways of eating have over ketogenic diets are their flexibility and increased sustainability. It's a whole lot easier to order low-carb options from a menu when you don't have to worry about being kicked out of ketosis!

A low-carb diet is generally considered to include between 100 and 150 grams of total carbs per day. Note that this is *not* net carbs, as low-carb diets don't tend to require the same intensity of macronutrient tracking that ketogenic diets do (although, if you love tracking, I won't stop you). While there are plenty of official low-carb diets out there under various patented names with rules and lists of allowable and forbidden foods, the kind of low-carb I'm talking about here is a more laid-back approach that focuses on eating foods that make you feel good.

Making the transition from keto to a general low-carb diet is relatively easy. You can pretty much keep eating the way you've been eating, but start making higher-carb additions and substitutions to your meals. For example, you could include more fruit and berries in your smoothies. Instead of cauliflower mash at dinner, maybe you start having sweet potato mash. As I mentioned previously, I generally suggest making changes slowly, such as modifying one meal at a time for a few days before adding more carbs, to see how your body reacts.

Check out pages 52 to 59 for suggestions of foods to incorporate into a low-carb diet.

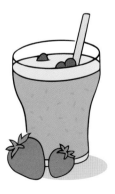

Transitioning to a Medium-Carb Diet

If a low-carb diet still seems a little too restrictive for you long term, might I suggest a medium-carb way of eating? I promise I'm not making things up just to sound cool or trendy. In fact, my friend actually came up with this term, and I really, really like it. *Medium-carb* is a great way to describe a way of eating that isn't quite low-carb, but also isn't the typical high-carb diet that most of us started out on.

Basically, a medium-carb diet is to the low-carb and keto sphere what a flexitarian diet is to the vegetarian and vegan sphere. There's an emphasis on eating mostly low-carb foods as the base, but with higher-carb additions like sweet potatoes, legumes, fruit, and even grains/pseudograins. Tracking isn't really part of the deal, and "real" sweeteners like maple syrup and honey may even make appearances.

I like to think of a medium-carb way of eating as simply avoiding the highly processed sugary and carby foods that we find ourselves inundated with and instead eating whole foods that nourish our bodies. Ideally, the basis of most meals is still nonstarchy vegetables with fats and protein, but the addition of higher-carb plant foods is encouraged and in no way limited.

I've included lists of what I like to think of as medium-carb foods on pages 59 to 61, so you can add them in if you choose to make high-carb days a part of your routine, and to help you plan meals if you decide to transition off a ketogenic diet or want to start carb cycling.

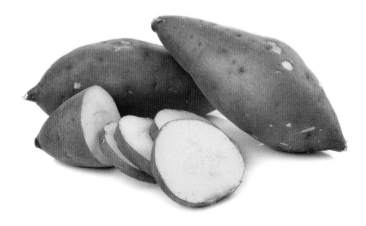

Finding Balance

It's important to note that you don't have to eat one way all the time. If you want to eat keto for three months and then low-carb for a month on a loop, you totally can. If you'd rather transition off keto to a generally low-carb way of eating and then eat a more medium-carb diet over the holidays, go for it! Low-carb and medium-carb ways of eating are general guidelines to help you find what works best for you in the long run, but how you eat is ultimately up to you and what feels best for your body.

One thing I've learned from trying to optimize my own approach to keto over the years is that our bodies are always changing and may need different things at different times. There's nothing wrong with modifying the way you eat to accommodate those changes.

Just remember, there are no hard-and-fast rules, and you don't have to keep doing something the same way if it isn't working for you!

Will I Gain Weight After Stopping Keto?

One of the most common anxieties I see echoed by my clients and across social media is the prospect of gaining weight after transitioning away from a ketogenic diet. This is a reasonable concern, especially for those who used keto for weight loss. After all, you have put in all this hard work, and you don't want to see your progress erased. Completely understandable!

When you transition off a ketogenic diet, you may notice a small (2- to 3ish-pound) weight bump as your muscles begin to store more glycogen and, with it, more water. This is basically just reversing that quick water-weight drop that people notice in the first few days of being in ketosis. This isn't fat gain, and it isn't something to stress about. Sometimes it evens out, sometimes not. But again, it's just water weight that comes with increased carbohydrate consumption.

Of course, I realize that the vast majority of people are not concerned with small fluctuations in weight. In fact, it's normal to notice some daily variance with or without keto, especially for those of us with menstrual cycles who are accustomed to gaining 2 to 5 pounds (and sometimes more) for around a week every month. This is one of the reasons that daily weigh-ins are typically not recommended!

Most people are more anxious about reversing their progress and putting back on all of the fat that they lost while in ketosis. From my own experience with keto and my years of working to get people on and off ketogenic diets as a nutritionist, I can say anecdotally that no, you do not automatically put back on all of the weight after stopping a ketogenic diet, especially if you continue eating a low- to medium-carb diet.

From what I've observed over the years, the people who gain weight back after stopping a ketogenic diet tend to have one thing in common: they go back to their old ways of eating. This is why I typically suggest finding a happy medium between the diet that brought you to keto and a ketogenic or very-low-carb diet.

This is also why I recommend transitioning off a ketogenic diet slowly, as you'll be able to recognize how certain foods impact you and work toward being able to eat intuitively.

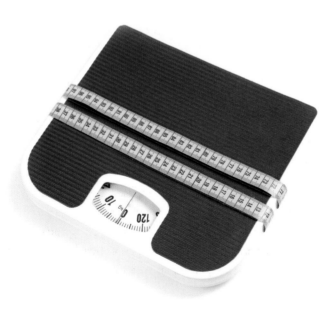

Eating Plants

Now that I've talked a bit about ketogenic diets, what a plant-forward ketogenic diet is, and all of the different ways you can follow a plant-forward ketogenic diet, let's move on to the star of the show: the plants. One of my favorite quotes of all time comes from a Michael Pollan book, *In Defense of Food.* He succinctly sums up what has become my guiding light when making food choices:

"Eat food. Not too much. Mostly plants."

The message is super simple and gets to the point. I also love this quote because you can apply it to nearly every style of eating out there. I'm not here to tell you to eat less meat, or to go vegan, or to eat only vegetables and get all your energy through photosynthesis. That's not my place. I'm also not here to preach at you that one way of eating is better than another. The mission of this book is simply to help you eat more awesome plant foods within the context of a ketogenic diet. So, let's talk about plants!

Nowadays, I'm a little bit obsessed with eating plants, but I definitely didn't start out that way. As a child, I remember turning my nose up at pretty much every healthy thing my mom put in front of me. Broccoli, cauliflower, turnips—no, no, and absolutely not. Even fruit was too healthy-tasting for me. After my mom would cut up a bowl of strawberries or an apple, I would sneak back into the kitchen and drown it in sugar. Thinking about that still makes me cringe a little bit.

As I got older, my tastes began to change. I learned to tolerate salads because they were low in calories and I thought they would help me lose weight. This was pretty much my view of vegetables throughout high school and even into college. I ate more vegetables than I had as a child, but it was somewhat begrudgingly and wholly motivated by my wanting to be thin.

It wasn't until Michael Pollan's *The Omnivore's Dilemma* hit bookstores that I really thought about vegetables and fruits as being an important part of my diet. That book opened my eyes to the world of food and nutrition outside the 1990s diet-crazed bounds of calories and fat. It was a revelation that led me to read so many more books about food, nutrition, and health and then eventually to enroll in a nutrition education program.

From there, not only did I learn about the health benefits of eating more vegetables, but I learned how to prepare them so that I actually *wanted* to eat them. And later, when I started experimenting with ketogenic diets, I also started eating more vegetables. After all, once I wasn't eating bread or pasta at every meal, I had to fill that void with something!

Why am I telling you all of this? Mostly because I want you to know that I am in no way judging those who don't eat vegetables. In fact, I basically didn't eat vegetables until my twenties, and then I didn't really eat anything beyond frozen peas and carrots (still a comfort food for me!) until I was about 25 and studying nutrition.

Of course, none of that explains why *you* should eat vegetables. In this section, we're going to talk about many of the nutritional benefits of including more plant foods in your diet, from the basics to a slightly deeper dive into the fascinating world of phytonutrients.

Three Great Reasons to Add More Plants to Your Plate

I'm always apprehensive about making a definitive statement on any particular point in the field of nutrition. We have learned so much over the past decade about how our genetics and environments play a key role in how we metabolize food to the point that it's reasonable to say we really are all different. Because I choose to eat a plant-based diet, I also worry that people will think I'm judging their food choices if they don't eat the same way. (I'm not!)

However, there are some areas of nutrition where I feel pretty confident in stating an opinion, and here is one of them: I think eating plants is good for you. Not groundbreaking, I know. I also know that there are people out there who have medical conditions that prevent them from eating loads of plants. But, for the vast majority of us, plants are beneficial foods.

Since you picked up this book, you likely don't need too much convincing on the eating plants front, but just in case, here are some basic reasons why it helps to increase your plant intake.

Plants Are Good for You

I'm going to start with a sentence you probably heard quite a bit growing up (and read in this book just thirty seconds ago): "They're good for you." It's no secret that fruits, vegetables, nuts, seeds, and beans are rich in vitamins and minerals, which our bodies need to function. Fruits and vegetables in particular deliver these nutrients along with a hefty dose of water, which can help us stay hydrated.

While many processed foods are fortified with vitamins and minerals, as I'll discuss in more detail a little later, plants contain many additional nutrients that work synergistically with vitamins and minerals to provide nutritional benefits that are greater than the sum of their parts.

Plants Are Delicious

I think we can all agree that fruit tastes amazing, but vegetables do, too! I used to think I hated a lot of vegetables. I grew up in the fat-phobic '90s, eating plain raw, steamed, or boiled vegetables without oil, butter, or even salt. For this reason, I thought I hated vegetables.

Fun fact: Adding some oil and seasoning (even just salt and/or pepper!) can make anything taste incredible. You may think you don't like kale, or broccoli, or Brussels sprouts...but I don't want you to jump to that conclusion without trying them roasted with some olive oil and seasoning. Vegetables bring so many textures and flavors to a meal, whether they're the main event, a side dish, or even just chopped up and snuck into a meatloaf (or a Beyond meatloaf, in my case).

Plants Fill You Up

I don't know about you, but I'm a volume eater. I love being able to chow down on a giant stir-fry or salad. Because of their high water and fiber content, vegetables tend to fill you up physically, stimulating the stretch receptors in your stomach and intestines[12] and signaling that you're full. This feeling of satiety is compounded by incorporating fats (the staple of a keto diet) into your meals.[13] A larger-volume meal should also take longer to eat than a calorically dense meal, and studies routinely show that eating meals a bit slower is beneficial to our digestive systems.[14]

Eat the Rainbow for More Nutrition

The nutritional benefits of plant foods don't end with their vitamin and mineral content. In fact, that barely scratches the surface. The more we study fruits, vegetables, nuts, and beans, the more we learn about their chemical makeup and how so many moving parts contribute to the nutritional benefits they convey.

You may have heard that you should "eat the rainbow" (not to be confused with "taste the rainbow") because different colors of fruits and vegetables have different nutritional benefits. While it sounds a little childish and reductive, there's a lot of merit to this line of thinking! The colors in plants are the result of their chemical makeup of various phytonutrients, and some of these colorful compounds offer up nutritional benefits to those who consume them.

Phytonutrients (or phytochemicals, as they're often called) are chemicals that give plants their colors, aromas, and flavors. These compounds serve many purposes within the plant, including regulating growth, fostering communication with other plants, and aiding in the plants' defense.[15] While phytochemicals are not essential to the human diet, consuming them has been shown to be quite beneficial. Studies have long demonstrated that eating a diet high in fruits and vegetables (upwards of 500 grams a day) is related to lower incidences of cardiovascular disease, certain cancers, and other chronic ailments,[16] and these positive benefits may be attributed in part to the phytochemical contents of the plants.

Scientists estimate that there are over 5,000 different phytochemicals, but as of writing this book, studies have been limited to a tiny fraction of these.[17] Even still, those that have been studied number far too many to cover here, so I'm just going to talk about the most common ones with the most research behind them.

It's important to note that cooking foods can destroy some of these beneficial phytochemicals (as well as some heat-sensitive vitamins), but it also destroys antinutrients that can inhibit mineral absorption and cause some digestive complications. Adding to the confusion, some nutrients, like lycopene, actually become more bioavailable when heated. So, in addition to recommending that you eat a wide variety of plant sources to diversify your phytochemical intake, I recommend eating both cooked and raw fruits and vegetables. It's all about balance.

While it's not a perfect model, I'm going to arrange these commonly studied phytonutrients by color because it's fun and because having a visual association helps me retain information better—I hope it helps you as well. I try to eat a well-rounded selection of vegetables from a few different color families each day to diversify the micronutrients and phytochemicals I'm eating. The rainbow visual helps me keep my meals from being entirely green and brown.

You will notice that there is a lot of overlap between groups, as individual plants contain many different phytochemicals, but I'm just going to list the most common sources of each. I've included some higher-carb fruits and vegetables in the following lists because I think they're worth mentioning. While it's true that you're probably not going to be able to eat a whole mango on a ketogenic diet and stay in ketosis, a 2-tablespoon serving of Trader Joe's mango salsa has 4 grams of net carbs, which could easily be worked into your macros from time to time, especially if you're eating at least 30 grams of net carbs per day.

I also want to point out that none of these lists is complete. I tried to focus on the most common sources of these particular phytochemicals (with some more interesting sources thrown in as well), but all fruits, vegetables, nuts, seeds, and beans contain phytonutrients.

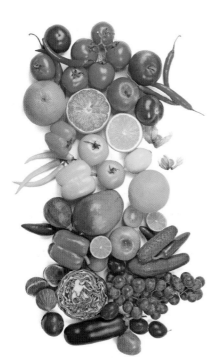

Do Animal Foods Have Phytochemicals?

Nope! Phytochemicals are found in plants and fungi (which are technically not plants) but are not produced by animals. The prefix *phyto-* comes from the Greek word for "plants," so when you see it at the start of a word, you can be sure the word is somehow plant-related. Animal foods have an equivalent to phytochemicals, called *zoochemicals*, which have not been studied quite as thoroughly as their plant counterparts but are gaining more attention.

Bright Reds: Lycopene

Red foods tend to be rich in lycopene, which studies have shown is one of the most powerful antioxidants among all of the dietary carotenoids. Consumption of lycopene-rich foods like tomatoes correlates with a decreased risk of cardiovascular disease and some types of cancer, including prostate and breast cancers.[18] Research is also being conducted on the potential protective nature of lycopene against cognitive decline[19] and metabolic syndrome.[20]

As I mentioned previously, lycopene becomes more bioavailable when cooked, so tomato sauce and tomato soup aren't just delicious and comforting; they're also loaded with bioavailable lycopene.

The fruit most commonly associated with lycopene (and the focus of so many of these studies) is the tomato, but there are several other notable sources.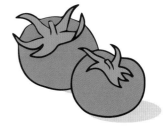

Food sources: tomatoes, goji berries, papaya, pink grapefruit, pink guava, watermelon

Dark Red, Purple, Blue & Black: Anthocyanins

Anthocyanins are the pigments in plant foods that impart dark red, purple, blue, and black hues. These phenols have been studied for many health effects, including their antioxidant and antimicrobial properties, as well as the ability to improve visual and neurological health[21] and aid in the prevention of cardiovascular disease, metabolic disorders, and even certain cancers.[22]

Interestingly, one of the highest concentrations of dietary anthocyanins is found in the skin of black soybeans,[23] which happen to be super keto-friendly, having a very low carb count and a relatively high protein content. Black soybeans are the basis for many of those keto black bean noodles you see in the food aisle of T.J. Maxx (and the grocery store).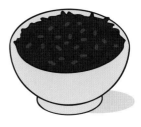

Food sources: blackberries, blueberries, black rice, black soybeans, cherries, concord grapes, cranberries, eggplant (in the peel), raspberries, red cabbage

Note: You may be thinking, "Where are the beets?"—and that would make sense. Beets are often a super dark purplish-red, so you'd think they'd be *loaded* with anthocyanins. Oddly enough, they don't contain any! Beets get their color from betalains, another phytochemical group that has been shown in studies to be protective against certain cancers, cognitive disorders, metabolic conditions, and cardiovascular disease.[24] So, while they may not contain any anthocyanins, they're still loaded with antioxidants (plus vitamins and minerals).

Orange & Yellow: Beta-Cryptoxanthin

While orange and yellow fruits and vegetables contain significant quantities of alpha- and beta-carotenes, I thought I'd focus on a slightly less-discussed member of the carotene group of phytonutrients: beta-cryptoxanthin. Like other carotenes, beta-cryptoxanthin is a precursor to vitamin A, an important nutrient for eye health, growth, and development, as well as immune function.[25] Beta-cryptoxanthin has also demonstrated antioxidant properties in studies, as well as the potential to decrease the risk for certain cancers.[26] Another interesting aspect of this phytochemical being studied is its ability to aid in bone recalcification, which could help prevent osteoporosis.[27]

Carotenes in general are being studied for their anti-cancer properties as well as their potential for therapeutic applications in neurodegenerative diseases like Alzheimer's and Parkinson's.[28]

Carotene absorption in humans (and subsequent conversion to vitamin A) is improved by eating fat with carotene-rich foods. Lucky for us, that's pretty much what plant-forward keto is all about!

Food sources: cantaloupe, carrots, mangoes, papaya, pumpkin and winter squash, sweet potatoes

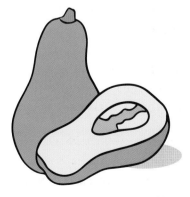

Yellow & Light Green: Lutein

Like lycopene and beta-cryptoxanthin, lutein is a carotenoid. This one imparts a yellowish color to fruits and vegetables (the word *lutein* comes from the Latin word *luteus*, which means "yellow"), though it can appear orange in high concentrations. Most of what is known about lutein relates to its role in eye health and its potential for preventing cataracts, diabetic retinopathy, and age-related macular degeneration, among other diseases.[29]

More recently, researchers are discovering that lutein may be beneficial for cognitive health at all ages as well. Lutein, like the other phytochemicals we've looked at, has both anti-inflammatory and antioxidant properties.[30]

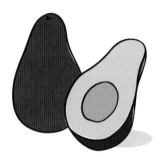

Food sources: avocado, corn, greens, kale, kiwi, marigold, nasturtium, peas, pistachios

Green: Sulforaphane

Sulforaphane has received a lot of attention from the nutrition community in the past few years for its promising anti-cancer effects,[31] but studies have suggested that it may have a beneficial effect on a whole constellation of conditions, including neurodevelopmental disorders, neurodegenerative diseases, cardiovascular disease, metabolic disorders, and liver disorders.[32] Each time a new study emerges, it seems to increase the potential for health benefits from consuming sulforaphane.

Interestingly, sulforaphane doesn't exist in the plant, but rather is converted from its precursor by the act of cleaving the molecule—most commonly by chewing. Broccoli is the most-studied source of this compound, but it is found in abundance in all cruciferous vegetables. To read more about cruciferous vegetables, check out page 72.

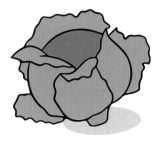

Food sources: broccoli, Brussels sprouts, cabbage, kale

What About White & Brown Foods?

I know we normally talk about white foods as being somewhat devoid of nutrition, but this is in the context of white sugar and flour, which have been heavily processed and stripped of most of the micronutrients present in the whole foods. White vegetables, on the other hand, are quite nutritious. Cauliflower isn't just adored for its versatility in the world of carb substitutes—it's also a nutrition powerhouse!

Many polyphenols (a type of phytochemical) don't have a color at all, so, while a plant may be a rich source of nutrients, they're not as visible as carotenes or anthocyanins. One phytonutrient present in white foods is allicin, which has demonstrated remarkable antimicrobial properties as well as the ability to reduce cholesterol and blood pressure.[33]

Another well-studied phytonutrient commonly found in white plant foods is quercetin, a flavonoid that has demonstrated anti-inflammatory, anti-cancer, and antiviral properties.[34] Quercetin is also being researched for its potential to reduce blood pressure[35] as well as potential anti-diabetic properties.[36]

White and tan foods also contain beneficial compounds like kaempferol, glucosinolates, and indoles. So, there's no reason to avoid white fruits and vegetables in the name of nutrient density!

Food sources: cauliflower, garlic, mushrooms, onions, potatoes, radishes

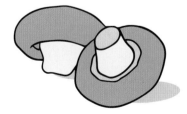

Further Reading

Phytonutrient interactions in plants and their nutritional benefits are such fascinating subjects, and there are so many studies underway now that it's impossible to mention everything in one book. If anything in this section piqued your interest, I highly recommend checking out the links in the endnotes. I also recommend heading over to PubMed (pubmed. ncbi.nlm.nih.gov) and checking out whatever studies interest you most. There are so many full-text studies available for browsing!

How Many Plants Do I Have to Eat?

This is kind of a tricky question. When I was growing up, I was told that five servings of fruits and vegetables was ideal. Now, new numbers are being thrown around every day. As with everything else, I think the ideal number of vegetables to eat in a day is the most you can tolerate. Ideally, at least according to a meta-analysis of 142 articles from 95 population studies,[37] we all should be eating at least 800 grams of fruit and vegetables per day. That's about 1.8 pounds, which roughly equates to eight servings.

If that seems like a lot, that's because it is for most of us. According to the Centers for Disease Control (CDC), only 9 percent of adults in the United States are eating the recommended five servings of fruits and vegetables per day.[38] I think it's important to point out that this isn't because we all hate eating vegetables. Many socioeconomic factors are at play, which could fill several very long books, that prevent many people from acquiring and/or affording an "adequate" (per the CDC) quantity of vegetables.

While eight servings of fruit and vegetables per day is certainly aspirational, the recommended five servings (around 500 grams) is a good place to start.

Can't I Just Take a Pill?

Yes and no. This is one of those situations where the sum is greater than the parts. Studies have shown that supplementation of individual micronutrients (lycopene and carotenoids are most often studied in this context) is not only less effective than consuming the whole food but can even be detrimental to health.[40] We really don't yet know how all of these compounds interact to produce the desired protective effects. So, taking any of them in isolation may not have any beneficial effect—and could even be harmful.

That being said, there are supplements made from whole foods, like greens powders (made from mostly green vegetables) and reds powders (made from red and purple vegetables and fruits), as well as multivitamins that are made from dehydrated fruits, vegetables, mushrooms, and other plants, that provide the whole spectrum of phytonutrients as they exist in the plants. So, if you really want to take a supplement to make up for not eating lots of vegetables, your best bet is to go with one made from actual whole foods.

Of course, I'm still a big fan of obtaining these phytochemicals by eating lots of vegetables and some fruit, with the exception of vitamins B_{12} and D, which are worth talking to your doctor about.

What About Antinutrients?

So far, I've only talked about the positive aspects of eating plant foods. However, as with most things in life, there is a balance. This is because not all phytochemicals have a protective or positive effect on our bodies. That would make things way too simple! I'll talk a little bit about how to mitigate the negative impact that antinutrients can have.

You may have heard mention of phytates, oxalates, and lectins, just to name a few of the most commonly discussed antinutrients. Some antinutrients are pro-inflammatory, while others can bind to nutrients and prevent your body from absorbing them properly. The good news is that there are some easy preparation methods that can help reduce or eliminate these compounds from food. Soaking, sprouting, fermenting, cooking, and especially pressure-cooking foods all reduce the concentration of various antinutrients. These methods are typically most successful when used in combination—for example, soaking and then cooking greens or soaking and then sprouting nuts or seeds.

If soaking, sprouting, fermenting, or pressure-cooking seems like it's adding too much work to your plate, then don't worry about it! Soaking and sprouting definitely take extra time and can be too much, especially if you're transitioning to a plant-forward way of eating. These preparation methods are just worth noting and perhaps keeping in mind if/when you have a little more time in the kitchen and want to maximize the nutritional benefit of your food.

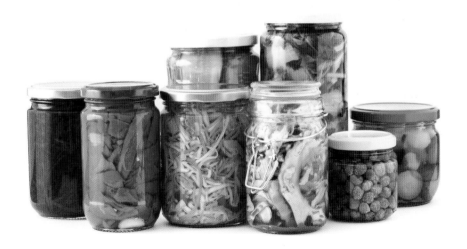

The Plant-Forward Keto Kitchen

I've talked a lot about why plants are so good for you, but I haven't really talked about which plants are ideal for plant-forward keto. Like I mentioned before, there are no "forbidden" foods on keto, nor is there a list of foods you *have* to eat to stay in ketosis. That said, it can be helpful to know which foods are lower in carbohydrates and therefore are likely to make up the bulk of your meals.

In this section, I'll talk about the many different types of plant foods you can incorporate into a plant-forward keto diet, especially plant-based proteins. (You don't have to rely on protein powder if you don't want to!) I'll also discuss some of the less common ingredients that are used in some of the recipes. And, for a quick reference, there are lists of low-carb plant foods, as well as some medium-carb foods, for those looking to employ carb cycling or transition away from a ketogenic diet.

Plant-Based Protein Sources

Tofu

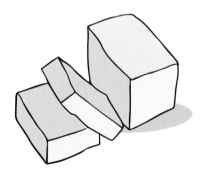

This will likely come as a surprise to absolutely no one, but tofu is a great source of protein. I know it has been the subject of a lot of scrutiny over the past few years due to the phytoestrogen content of soy, particularly by Paleo and other ancestral health movements, but I'm still a big fan of this protein powerhouse, at least in moderation.

I find that my digestive system tolerates sprouted tofu best, so that's usually what I buy. As a bonus, it's also lower in carbs than unsprouted tofu, and the two types cost about the same at Trader Joe's, where I often shop.

For those who can't eat soy but still want to eat tofu-based dishes, there are a *ton* of soy-free tofu options on the market now, and not just at specialty grocery stores or hippie co-ops! I've seen hemp tofu and pumpkin seed tofu at my regular grocery store, in the same section as the soy tofu and mock meats. While these soy-free alternatives are currently a bit expensive, I hope the prices will even out as they become more commonplace.

Tempeh

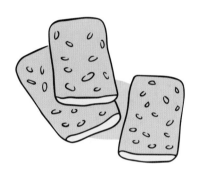

Like tofu, tempeh is a soy-based protein made from fermented soybeans. It is much firmer than tofu but can be sliced or crumbled. There are many different varieties of tempeh, including soy-free ones made from various beans, seeds, and nuts; my favorite is "hempeh," made from hemp seeds. It is worth noting that many types of tempeh are made with grains, so it's important to look at the nutrition label for the carb count if you are sticking with strict keto.

Nuts & Seeds

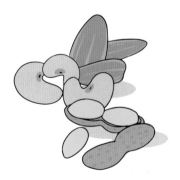

While most nuts and seeds aren't significant sources of protein, they do contain enough protein to be worth mentioning here. I usually eat two to three servings (a serving is typically 1 ounce/28g) of nuts and seeds every day, which provides a surprising portion of my protein.

Usually, I eat nuts by themselves as a snack, though I often use them as a garnish when I want a meal to have a little more texture. Seeds, on the other hand, are usually a topping or included in recipes (like the flax crepes on page 96).

The following table lists some of the more common higher-protein low-carb nuts and seeds and their basic nutrition information.

Nut or Seed	Net Carbs Per 1 Ounce/28g	Protein Per 1 Ounce/28g
Pecans	1.2g	2.6g
Walnuts	2g	4.3g
Pumpkin seeds (shelled)	2.3g	8.5g
Hemp seeds*	2.4g	9.5g
Almonds	2.6g	6g
Sunflower seeds (shelled)	3.2g	5.9g
Peanuts**	4.2g	7g
Pistachios (shelled)	4.7g	5.7g
Cashews	7.6g	5.2g

Data from the USDA's FoodData Central: https://fdc.nal.usda.gov

*Hemp seed numbers are based on 30g rather than 28g.

**While peanuts are technically legumes, not nuts, I have included them here because we tend to eat them the same way.

Note: These numbers are for raw nuts and seeds. Keep in mind that roasting them will reduce their moisture content and change the amount of carbs by weight.

Nutritional Yeast

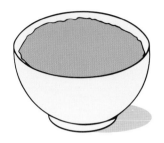

This is one of my favorite ways to add protein to a savory meal. Nutritional yeast (which is different from baker's yeast and brewer's yeast) is not only high in protein but also a great source of many B vitamins. Some brands are also fortified with B_{12}.

Nutritional yeast has a "cheesy" sort of flavor that can make dairy-free versions of recipes taste a little closer to their original inspiration. I like to blend nutritional yeast into sauces and use it in savory baked goods, but I also sprinkle it on veggies and noodle dishes for a little extra protein and flavor.

Protein Powders

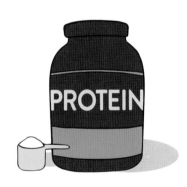

The easiest way to sneak protein into your meals on any diet is protein powder. It can be blended into smoothies, incorporated into baked goods, or simply mixed with water or nondairy milk for an easy shake.

There are many brands of plant-based protein powder out there that are sugar-free and keto-friendly. Many are also fortified with vitamins and minerals. Some even have additions like greens powders, adaptogens, mushroom powders, and MCT oil powder. For a list of some of my favorites, check out page 57.

Mock Meats, Dairy & Eggs

When I first went vegetarian back in the late 1990s, the selection of vegetarian meat substitutes on the market was limited. While you could find tofu pretty easily, mock meats were a whole different story. It wasn't until around the year 2000 that my local grocery stores started stocking a certain brand of fake burgers and chicken nuggets. So, in addition to tofu and some homemade seitan (which I ate when I was unaware that I had celiac disease, but now avoid because it is wheat-based), I ate a lot of Buffalo "chik'n" nuggets.

I also ate cheese and eggs back then, which was convenient because my local grocery stores definitely did not have plant-based versions of either of those foods.

The market has since exploded with plant-based alternatives to not only meat but dairy and eggs as well. And they can be found in regular grocery stores: you no longer have to trek to a natural grocery store to find these types of products (unless you want to, of course!). I've provided a list of some brands to look for on page 59.

Low-Carb Vegetable Swaps

Which vegetables should you eat instead of carb-heavy starches and grains? Now that keto has been trending for quite some time, there are loads of convenience foods on the market to replace high-carb staples in pretty much all of our meals. While these options are great, they're often expensive and don't really add much, nutritionally speaking. So, while I do enjoy these products from time to time, I mostly rely on the following simple vegetable swaps to replace carbs when adapting a non-keto recipe.

Note: Vegetables marked with a (c) are on the higher end of the carb spectrum but can still fit into a ketogenic diet.

Rice

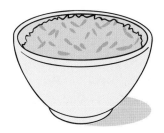

Cauliflower isn't the only vegetable you can rice! I also take broccoli stalks, peel off the harder bits, and blitz them through the food processor to make broccoli rice. You can rice beets (c) and carrots (c) as well, though, due to their carb count, I tend to mix them in with riced cauliflower or broccoli instead of using them on their own (like in my Rainbow Veggie Pilaf on page 214).

Noodles

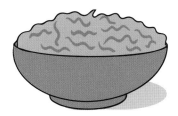

While zucchini noodles seem to get all of the attention, many other vegetables can be used to make noodles. Summer squash, carrots (c), beets (c), and radishes can be spiral-sliced. Roasted spaghetti squash (c) is another great alternative to pasta. You can even julienne hearts of palm to make a surprisingly good noodle.

My favorite low-carb veggie noodle is cabbage noodles. I like to cut thin strips of cabbage and sauté them in a little olive oil and salt until tender, then use them in place of noodles. If the cabbage noodles are being used in a soup, you don't even need to cook them before tossing them into the pot!

There is also an absolute *ton* of keto-friendly premade noodles available at most grocery stores today. Black soybeans (and other beans), almond flour, cauliflower, spaghetti squash, and hearts of palm all form the basis for store-bought low-carb noodles. And don't forget the shirataki (konjac) and kelp noodles that have been making appearances in keto recipes for the past decade or so.

Roasted Potatoes

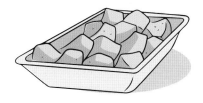

Since rice and noodles are often just vehicles for sauce or delicious toppings, it's relatively easy to replace them with vegetables and not miss the real thing too much. Roasted potatoes have always presented a somewhat harder challenge, as they're the actual focal point and not just a carrier. These substitutions won't make you forget that potatoes ever existed, but they are darn tasty in their own right. After peeling and cubing, the following lower-carb vegetables can be roasted in the exact same way you would roast potatoes: celeriac, kohlrabi, radishes, butternut squash (c), and kabocha squash (c).

Mashed Potatoes

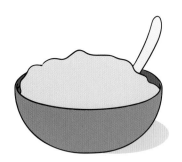

I've always felt that what made mashed potatoes so good wasn't necessarily the potatoes as much as the fats and salt. With that in mind, when adequately mashed (with minimal chunks!), seasoned, and oiled/buttered, the following vegetables mash up deliciously: broccoli, cauliflower, celeriac, kohlrabi, butternut squash (c), and kabocha squash (c).

Low-Carb Plant Foods

The lists that follow do not contain every keto-friendly plant food out there, but they're a good place to start. I've primarily listed foods that are common in North American grocery stores, though some may be available only seasonally (for instance, dandelion greens are only available in my local grocery stores in the springtime). I've also included some less-common ingredients (pili nuts, for example) that can be found from online health food retailers and in health food stores.

I've also chosen to include only whole foods and simple ingredients (like shirataki noodles and mustard), omitting prepackaged keto snack products, as there are so many new items coming to market every day that it's impossible to keep track of them all. That doesn't mean that you can't eat prepackaged snacks, though!

Note: Foods marked with a (p) are good sources of protein, and foods marked with a (c) are a bit higher in carbs and will likely have to be moderated depending on your carb target.

Fats

Nuts

Almonds (p)

Brazil nuts

Cashews (c)

Hazelnuts (also called filberts)

Macadamia nuts

Peanuts (I know they're technically legumes…)

Pecans

Pili nuts

Pine nuts (c)

Pistachios (c)

Walnuts

Seeds

Chia seeds

Flax seeds

Hemp seeds (p)

Pumpkin seeds (pepitas) (p)

Sacha inchi seeds (p)

Sunflower seeds (p)

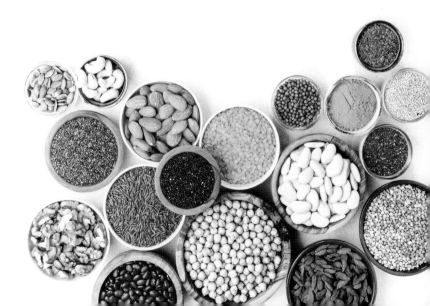

Nut & Seed Butters

Almond butter (p)

Coconut butter (coconut manna)*

Hazelnut butter

Macadamia nut butter

Peanut butter (p)

Pecan butter

Pili nut butter

Sunflower seed butter

Tahini

Walnut butter

Coconut butter (or manna) is sometimes referred to as creamed coconut but is completely different from coconut cream. Coconut butter/manna/creamed coconut is ground-up dried coconut, whereas coconut cream is ground-up fresh coconut, often with added water.

Other Whole-Food Fat Sources

Avocados

Coconut

Olives

Healthy Oils

Almond oil (also great for body care)

Avocado oil

Cacao butter (great for desserts and body care)

Coconut oil

Flaxseed oil (not for cooking; store in a cool, dark place)

Hazelnut oil

Macadamia nut oil

MCT oil (for adding to smoothies, coffee, and so on)

Olive oil

Walnut oil

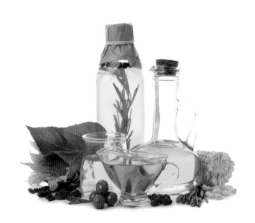

Low-Carb Vegetables

Artichoke hearts

Arugula

Asparagus

Beets (c)

Bell peppers (green are the lowest in carbs)

Bok choy

Broccoli

Broccoli rabe/raab/rapini

Brussels sprouts (c)

Cabbage

Carrots (c)

Cauliflower

Celeriac (also called celery root) (c)

Celery

Chard

Collards

Cucumbers

Daikon

Dandelion greens

Eggplant

Endive

Fennel

Fiddleheads (available for a short time in spring)

Garlic

Jicama

Kale

Kohlrabi

Lettuce (all types)

Mushrooms

Mustard greens

Okra

Onions (c)

Parsnips (c)

Radishes

Rhubarb

Rutabaga (c)

Shallots

Snow peas

Spinach

Squash, winter (butternut, pumpkin, spaghetti) (c)

Squash, yellow

Swiss chard

Tomatoes

Turnips

Zucchini

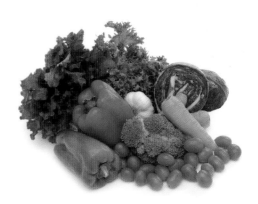

Low-Carb Fruits

Avocado

Coconut

Cranberries (fresh or frozen, not dried)

Lemons

Limes

Olives

Raspberries

Strawberries

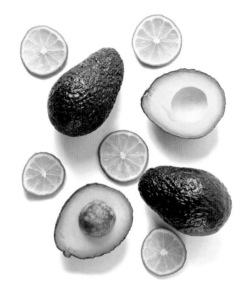

Pantry Items

Artichoke hearts

Baking powder

Baking soda

Black soybean noodles (c)

Black soybeans

Chocolate, dark (85 percent and up is usually super low in sugar, but be sure to check labels)

Cocoa or cacao powder

Coconut flour

Coconut milk (canned full-fat)

Hearts of palm

Herbs and spices, dried

Jackfruit, green (canned in brine, not syrup)

Kelp flakes

Kelp noodles

Lupin flour or soy flour (p)

Lupini beans (jarred in brine) (p)

Nori sheets

Nut and seed butters

Nut and seed flours

Nutritional yeast (p)

Psyllium husks (whole husks tend to work better than powder for baking)

Seaweed snacks

Vanilla extract (check for added sugar!)

Fridge Items

Cheese substitutes, dairy-free

Edamame (p)

Microgreens and sprouts

Milk, nondairy

Pickles, dill or other sugar-free type

Sauerkraut or vegan kimchi

Seitan (if not gluten intolerant)
(c) (p)

Shirataki noodles

Tempeh (p)

Tofu (p)

Yogurt, dairy-free, unsweetened (c)

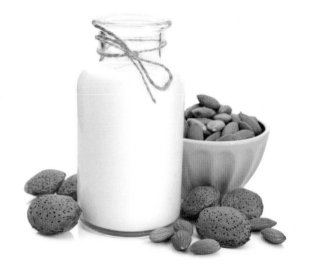

Protein Powders

Note: This list is far from exhaustive, especially as new protein powders are introduced to the market pretty much daily. This is just a list of plant-based, keto-friendly protein powders that I have tried and feel comfortable recommending. These particular brands are relatively easy to find and use high-quality ingredients. Some are sweetened, some are not, so be sure to check the labels!

Any unsweetened, single-ingredient protein powder (such as pea protein powder, rice protein powder, or soy protein isolate)

Garden of Life Raw

Legion Plant+

Manitoba Harvest Hemp Yeah!

Navitas Organics Essential Superfood Blend

Nutiva Hemp Seed Protein

Sunwarrior Classic Plus

Sunwarrior Warrior Blend

Vega Clean Protein

Vega Protein & Energy

Vega Sport Protein

Beverages

Coffee

Seltzer water

Tea (all kinds, as long as it doesn't contain sugar)

Water (mineral water is great for electrolytes)

Small servings of fermented beverages like kombucha, water kefir, and kvass (be sure to find low-sugar varieties)

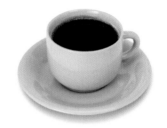

Creamers for Coffee & Tea

Coconut milk, canned full-fat

Coconut milk, powdered

Nondairy milk, unsweetened

Other creamers marketed toward keto diets*

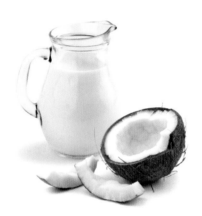

These products are tasty and keto-friendly, but keep in mind that despite what companies and influencers will have you believe, it is totally not necessary to buy or consume them!

Mock Meats & Other Plant-Based Foods

There are many mock meat brands on the market, with more being introduced all the time. It is important to look at the nutrition labels, as many mock meats are surprisingly high in carbohydrates. Here are a few of my favorite lower-carb options that are relatively widely available.

Beyond Meat products (burgers, meatballs, sausages, ground meat, and more)

Dr. Praeger's All American Burger

Dr. Praeger's Perfect Burger

Gardein: some products*

Impossible products (burgers, ground meat)

Quorn: some products*

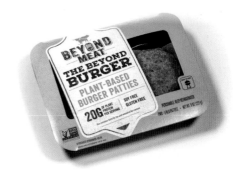

While Gardein and Quorn produce many different products, some are breaded and therefore higher in carbs. Additionally, some Quorn products contain eggs, so if you are looking to avoid eggs entirely, definitely check the ingredients!

Medium-Carb Plant Foods

This list is intended as a jumping-off point for incorporating slightly higher-carb foods into your meals—either for carb cycling or for transitioning from a ketogenic diet to a general low-carb or medium-carb diet. While there are no forbidden foods on keto, it would be pretty difficult to work many of these foods into a ketogenic meal plan on a regular basis, or at least in any appreciable quantity. That being said, I do manage to fit regular hummus and blueberries into a ketogenic diet pretty often, so your mileage may vary.

These foods can easily be worked into the recipes and meal plans in this book (or your favorite low-carb recipes) to transition from a ketogenic diet. Of course, this list is in no way complete, and just because a food doesn't appear here doesn't mean it isn't "allowed" on a medium-carb diet or in the context of carb cycling. In fact, foods being allowed (or not) is antithetical to the whole concept. You can eat whatever you want to increase your carb count; this list is just meant to give you some whole-food plant-based inspiration.

Note: These foods are deemed to be medium-carb per average serving, not necessarily for an entire piece of fruit—I'm mostly thinking about pineapple, bunches of grapes, and giant sweet potatoes that are the size of your head.

Fruits

Apples

Apricots

Blueberries

Cherries

Grapefruit

Grapes

Kiwis

Mandarins

Melon (cantaloupe, honeydew, watermelon)

Oranges

Pears

Pineapple

Beans

Black beans

Chickpeas

Great Northern beans

Navy beans

Pinto beans

Red kidney beans

Vegetables

Bell peppers

Corn

Green beans

Peas

Potatoes

Squash, winter (acorn, kabocha, delicata)

Sugar snap peas

Sweet potatoes

Taro root

Beverages

Kombucha and other fermented beverages

Oat milk

Rice milk

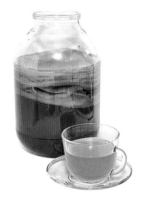

Pantry Items

Bean dips and salads

Bean pastas (black bean, chickpea, lentil, mung bean, and so on)

Lentil and bean soups

Oatmeal

Popcorn

Potato chips

Quinoa and quinoa flour

Fridge Items

Hummus (all kinds!)

Ketchup, sauces, and dressings (low-sugar)

Yogurt (low-sugar)

Freezer Items

Bean burgers

All mock meats (even the breaded ones!)

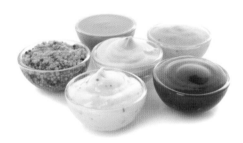

Special Ingredients

Because ketogenic and low-carb diets tend to include some unusual foods, I thought I'd provide descriptions of some of the less-common grocery items used in this book.

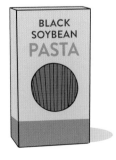

Black Soybean Pasta

I've mentioned this pasta a few times, and it's because I eat black soybean noodles pretty frequently. They're relatively low in carbs and high in fiber and protein. I also like the texture of the noodles far better than any other low-carb replacement, and that's worth the extra carbs to me.

Black soybean noodles are pretty widely available—I've found them everywhere from my regular grocery store to the food section of HomeGoods, plus many online retailers (including Amazon and Thrive Market). There are a lot of different brands out there, and they tend to have roughly similar macros. A few brands are marketed as "black bean noodles" instead of "black soybean noodles," so check the ingredients to be sure, as regular black beans are far higher in carbohydrates.

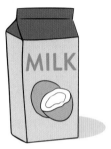

Coconut Milk

Two types of coconut milk are available in most grocery stores: unsweetened coconut milk and full-fat canned coconut milk. These two varieties have vastly different water and fat contents and cannot be used interchangeably.

Unsweetened coconut milk is the thinner variety that you find in cartons in the dairy aisle, as well as in the cereal aisle with the other nondairy milks. Unsweetened coconut milk can be used in any recipe in this book that calls for nondairy milk.

Full-fat canned coconut milk is, as the name says, canned and can often be found in a few different places in the grocery store. I have seen it with the shelf-stable nondairy milks, in the baking aisle near the condensed milk and evaporated milk, and with the Thai specialty foods. Typically, there are two types of canned coconut milk: full-fat (often just labeled *coconut milk*) and light/lite. The light variety is lower in fat and has a higher water content, which makes it a great coffee creamer, but I tend to use the full-fat version in recipes.

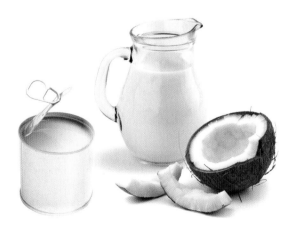

Coconut Cream

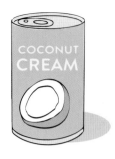

If you have an incredibly well-stocked grocery store, you may see canned coconut cream. Coconut cream is even denser than full-fat canned coconut milk, with very little liquid. It makes a great frosting when whipped, as well as a great mousse when combined with other ingredients. You can also make your own coconut cream by chilling a can of full-fat coconut milk overnight and scooping out the cream that solidifies on top of the liquid. (Discard or compost the liquid from the bottom of the can, or use it in smoothies.) You can get about 1 cup (240ml) cream from a 13.5-ounce (400-ml) can of coconut milk. The cream will keep in an airtight container in the refrigerator for up to 5 days.

Coconut Oil

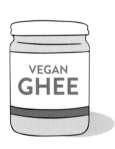

I pretty much exclusively use unrefined, cold-pressed coconut oil in cooking and baking, unless I really don't want whatever I'm cooking to taste like coconut. Cold-pressed, unrefined oils retain far more of their nutrients and phytochemicals and have more flavor.

If you don't want your recipes to taste too coconutty, you can use refined coconut oil. There are also refined coconut oils on the market that have a more buttery taste. The one I use most is Nutiva's vegan ghee, which is a blend of coconut and avocado oils.

Flaxseed, Ground

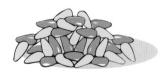

I have listed ground flaxseed separately from nut and seed flours because while technically it is ground-up seeds, ground flax is typically used as a binder and not as a flour. I prefer to grind my own flax seeds as needed because flax oils are fairly delicate and can go rancid quickly when exposed to light, heat, or oxygen.

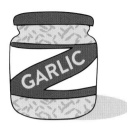

Garlic, Minced

I usually use a garlic press or Microplane grater to make my garlic nice and smooth, but you can also smash and then finely mince the clove. If you really dislike mincing garlic (or just don't want to deal with it), you can also use the jarred kind from the store. I tend to keep one of those on hand, because sometimes I have zero desire to clean a garlic press.

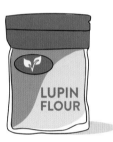

Lupin Flour (aka Lupini Bean Flour)

Lupin flour, like other bean flours, is made of ground-up beans (lupini beans, in this case; see below). Lupin flour is really high in protein and fiber and really low in carbs, making it a perfect choice for keto and low-carb baking.

I love using lupin flour in recipes because, like chickpea flour, it works really well as a replacement for all-purpose wheat flour, especially in crusts and cookies.

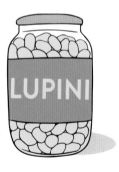

Lupini Beans (Lupins)

These beans are super high in protein and low in carbs, and stories say they were consumed by Roman soldiers and Egyptian pharaohs alike. Lupins are extremely bitter, so a weeklong brining process is required to make them palatable. For this reason, I prefer to buy them jarred in brine instead of dried.

Lupini beans are sold in jars, not in cans like many other prepared beans. Typically, I find the jars in the Mediterranean, Latin American, and kosher sections of grocery stores.

Allergen note: There is some cross-reactivity between lupini beans and peanuts, so you may want to avoid them if you have a peanut allergy.

Quality is very important here, though. Lupini flour should not taste super bitter. If it does, the beans were not soaked long enough before being dried and ground. I have tried the Lopina brand many times, and each time it has been delicious! If you are looking for a lower-cost option, soy flour can replace lupin flour. Chickpea flour can also replace lupin flour but is a bit higher in carbohydrates.

Allergen note: There is some cross-reactivity between lupini beans and peanuts, so you may want to avoid lupin flour if you have a peanut allergy.

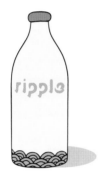

Milks, Nondairy

If you've gone to a grocery store lately, you may have noticed the wild explosion of nondairy milks available. While any nondairy milk can be used in these recipes, those made from coconut, nuts, and seeds are typically the lowest in carbs. I also really like pea milk (the brand I buy is Ripple) and soy milk, as both are high in protein.

Be sure to buy the unsweetened varieties, and make sure you know what flavor the milk is. That may sound silly, but the first time I tried to make macaroni and "cheeze" from scratch, I didn't realize I had bought vanilla soy milk...it was not great.

Typically, grocery stores stock nondairy milks in two sections—the refrigerated area, right next to the dairy case, and the cereal aisle, where the milks can be found in shelf-stable packaging.

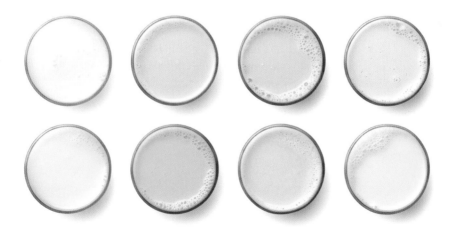

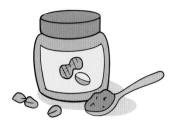

Nut & Seed Butters

The nut and seed butters I use in my recipes are the ones typically labeled *natural* with only two ingredients: nuts/seeds and salt. This is important to note; oftentimes additional oils are added to commercial nut butters, which can change their texture and alter the outcome of a recipe.

Because I use nut and seed butters so often, I keep them at room temperature so they're always ready to use in a recipe. If you prefer to keep your nut and seed butters in the fridge, be sure to give them enough time to come up to room temperature before trying to measure them.

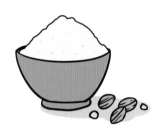

Nut & Seed Flours

Flours made from nuts and seeds are used liberally in keto, low-carb, and gluten-free baking.

For the most part, nut and seed flours are interchangeable. If you cannot tolerate almond flour, for example, hazelnut flour or sunflower seed flour will work in its place. The flavor of the finished recipe will be slightly different, but this is not an issue in many baked goods, where additional flavors are present and tend to mask the taste of the flour.

Note that nut meals and nut flours are different. Nut meals are coarser, and the skins of the nuts remain. Nut flour is quite finely ground, and the skins are typically removed before the nuts are ground into flour.

I like to grind my own nut/seed meals and flours because it takes about 5 minutes and can cost up to 50 percent less than buying premade nut and seed flours. Plus, grinding my own nuts and seeds yields a fresher flour.

Nutritional Yeast

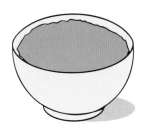

As I mentioned previously when talking about my favorite superfoods, I like nutritional yeast because it is incredibly nutrient-dense. It's relatively low in carbs and calories and high in protein and B vitamins. Nutritional yeast is actually the same variety as brewer's yeast and baker's yeast (*Saccharomyces cerevisiae*), but the yeast is inactivated during processing, so it can't be used to make beer or bread.

Nutritional yeast gives dishes a sort-of-cheesy, sort-of-nutty flavor. You'll notice I use it a lot in recipes, but I also sprinkle (okay, pour) it on top of roasted or sautéed vegetables, soups, noodles, and pretty much anything to which you could imagine adding grated cheese.

Olive Oil

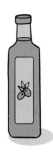

I typically buy cold-pressed, extra-virgin olive oil for cooking and making dressings. *Extra-virgin* just means that the oil came from the first pressing of the olives, so it retains the most nutrients and phytochemicals from the olives.

Be sure to buy olive oil in a dark-colored bottle and store it in a cool, dark place.

Protein Powder

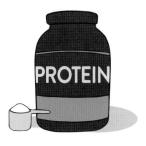

You'll notice that I don't specify a particular type of protein powder in many of the recipes, and that's because you can use pretty much any type of sugar-free protein powder you like.

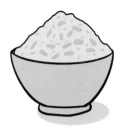

Psyllium Husk

This may seem like a weird ingredient, but you're likely more familiar with it than you realize! Typically, psyllium husk is sold as a digestive aid and fiber supplement; it's the main ingredient in those orange-flavored fiber drinks. In these recipes, it's used as a binder.

Psyllium husk is sold in whole husk form as well as a powder. I always use the whole husk form because I find that it clumps less, but if you have only the powder, that's okay, too. Just be sure to whisk it in thoroughly with the other ingredients. A teaspoon of psyllium husk powder is equivalent to a tablespoon of whole psyllium husks.

Plain psyllium husk is available in the gluten-free or health food aisle of many grocery stores and can often be found in the supplement section as well.

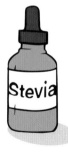

Salt

Those in ketosis tend to drink more water and flush out more electrolytes. To help offset this loss of electrolytes, I like to use either pink salt or Celtic sea salt, both of which contain trace minerals and electrolytes.

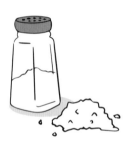

Sweeteners

There are so many sugar-free sweeteners out there now that trying to figure out which one to use, especially in a recipe, can get a little overwhelming and very confusing. While some sweeteners can replace full-sugar ones, others cannot, especially in baked goods, where sugar traditionally provides texture as well as sweetness.

The main sweeteners I use in these recipes (and in my daily life) are liquid stevia and granulated erythritol-based sweeteners. I also use sugar-free maple-flavored syrup, unflavored allulose syrup, and powdered sweetener on occasion.

For adding stevia to recipes, I prefer the unflavored liquid kind that you can find in many grocery store baking aisles. The brands I typically buy are the Whole Foods Market private label (365), NuNaturals, and NOW Foods. While some people prefer to use powdered stevia because it contains fewer ingredients, I like the liquid kind because it doesn't clump when mixed with other ingredients.

When it comes to granulated sweeteners, I like erythritol because it's usually the easiest to find. I also think it functions the most like sugar in recipes, and it's the gentlest on my digestive system. While many people like xylitol, I avoid it because it is highly toxic to pets; relatively small amounts can kill them.

While you can use plain erythritol, I tend to prefer varieties like Lakanto and Swerve that are blended with another sweetener to take the edge off of the cooling erythritol taste.

If you don't want to use sugar alcohols like erythritol and xylitol, allulose is another great option. Until recently, I had a difficult time finding it, so I'm always hesitant to recommend it over other options. Allulose is similar to erythritol in the way it functions in recipes, but it doesn't have that cool aftertaste.

The sugar-free maple syrup I like best is from Lakanto, and it is sweetened with a blend of monkfruit and erythritol, but there are plenty of other brands on the market. Just be aware that they all have different nutrition profiles.

Many of the companies that make granulated sweeteners also make confectioner's-style sweeteners, but if I just need a few tablespoons of that type, I tend not to buy a whole bag. To make your own powdered sweetener, just blitz your favorite granulated sweetener in a food processor or spice grinder.

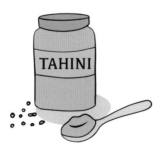

Tahini

Some brands and varieties of tahini are mild, while others have a distinct bitter flavor. I gravitate toward milder varieties and have had a lot of success with the private-label 365 tahini from Whole Foods Market, as well as those from the brands Levant and Once Again.

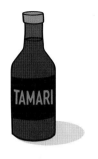

Tamari

Tamari is a Japanese soy sauce that is made without wheat and is thus gluten-free. Tamari tends to be darker and a bit less salty than traditional soy sauce. I typically use the low-sodium variety of tamari, which contains about one-third less sodium than regular varieties.

If you have a soy allergy, you can use coconut aminos in place of tamari or soy sauce, though coconut aminos is a bit sweeter and higher in carbs.

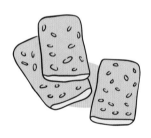

Tempeh

Made from fermented soybeans, tempeh is a nutrient-dense, low-carb plant protein. It has a firmer texture than tofu and a fairly distinct flavor. Tempeh can be found in most grocery stores alongside the tofu and other vegetarian foods. Be sure to read the labels, as some varieties of tempeh are made with grains and can be much higher in carbohydrates than others.

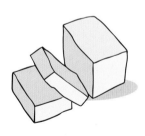

Tofu

Tofu is an incredibly versatile protein that absorbs flavor really well. The most important thing to note about buying tofu is that there are two main types: silken and firm/extra-firm. Silken tofu has a smooth texture and contains a lot of water. It makes a great base for puddings and pie fillings, as well as an egg replacer. Typically, you use silken tofu straight out of the package with no additional prep needed.

Firm (or extra-firm) tofu is, as the name implies, firmer and has less water content. This is the tofu to use when eating it on its own or in a stir-fry. Many people use a tofu press to get rid of excess moisture, but that's not required.

My favorite tofu trick is to freeze it in the package overnight and then thaw it (still in the package) before cooking. Once it has thawed, you can drain the liquid from the package and easily press out/squeeze out the remaining water by hand. This makes the tofu even firmer and prepares it well for baking or frying.

Nowadays, you can also find soy-free varieties like hemp tofu and pumpkin seed tofu at many grocery stores.

Four Groups of Superfoods You're (Probably) Already Eating

We hear the word *superfood* a lot, to the point where it kind of has no meaning anymore. And, while there certainly are foods that have a greater concentration of vitamins, minerals, and phytonutrients, you're probably already eating plenty of foods that are quite nutrient-dense and way more affordable.

Many of the so-called superfoods (goji berries, quinoa, chia seeds, moringa, açai, and maca, to name a few) that become media darlings place a strain on the growers, their land, and their communities, either by destroying the land due to overharvesting to meet international demand, by forcing farmers to divert resources away from growing other crops for their communities, or both. Additionally, most of the superfood berries, powders, and nuts on the market are sourced far from their target market, giving them a hefty carbon footprint.

That doesn't mean you have to give up that sprinkle of goji berries on top of your smoothie bowl if it really makes you happy, but there are loads of nutrient-dense foods that are much more affordable and generally lower in carbs. For the record, 1 tablespoon of dried goji berries has 3.7 grams of net carbohydrates, so it's not super low-carb, but if it's important to you...live your best life.

The term *superfood* simply refers to plant foods that have a higher nutrient density than others. Instead of focusing on trendy (and pricey) superfoods, I want to talk about very nutrient-dense plant foods that you're probably already eating. In fact, there's a good chance that you have a bunch of these in your fridge and pantry right now. These superfoods are not only easier to find, but they're also easier on the wallet.

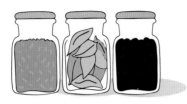

Herbs & Spices

I thought I'd start off easy with things that pretty much every one of us already has in the kitchen: herbs and spices. Many of these culinary staples were used as medicines long before they became simple food flavorings.[41]

Like fruits and vegetables, herbs and spices contain a plethora of antioxidant phytochemicals that work synergistically within the plant (and our bodies!).[42] These compounds also impart flavor and color.

Aside from the nutritional benefits, herbs and spices are a great way to add variety to your meals pretty affordably. While many spice blends seem a bit spendy when you look at the whole jar, it's usually a pretty minor expense when you break it down per serving.

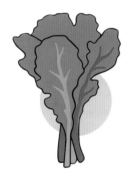

Cruciferous Vegetables

This is by far my favorite family of vegetables. Cruciferous (or brassica) vegetables are commonly referred to as the cabbage family, but cabbage is far from the only member. The most commonly consumed cruciferous vegetables are

- Arugula
- Bok choy
- Broccoli
- Brussels sprouts
- Cabbage
- Cauliflower
- Chard
- Collard and mustard greens
- Daikon radishes
- Horseradish
- Kale
- Kohlrabi
- Radishes
- Rapini (broccoli rabe)
- Rutabaga
- Turnips
- Wasabi
- Watercress

Odds are, you're already eating at least a few of these veggies somewhat regularly.

What makes this group of vegetables so great? Aside from the fact that they're loaded with fiber, protein, vitamins, and minerals, cruciferous vegetables contain a few phytochemicals that have somewhat excited the medical community. Several compounds in cruciferous plants currently being studied have shown promising antioxidant and anti-cancer properties.[43] One of these potentially cancer-preventing compounds that you may have heard of is sulforaphane,[44] which is found most abundantly in broccoli (particularly broccoli sprouts), Brussels sprouts, and bok choy.

In addition to their nutritional benefits, cruciferous vegetables add big flavor to dishes. I don't think I've ever encountered flavorless arugula or mustard leaves (not to mention wasabi and horseradish)! I'm also a big fan of the fact that it's a fairly affordable produce family as well. While some members might be a bit spendy, cabbage is wildly inexpensive.

Mushrooms

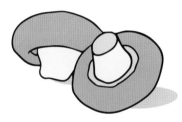

As I child, I *hated* mushrooms. I thought the texture was weird, the taste was weird—and they looked kind of weird, too. A big "no" from me all around. Of course, this was when I thought the only mushrooms out there were the kind that sit out for hours in grocery store salad bars, which is to say sadly droopy, raw, sliced button mushrooms. As I became a bit more adventurous with my food choices, I realized that there are loads of mushrooms out there, and they're all pretty delicious. While I'm still not sold on the idea of using a portobello cap as a burger, I've come to appreciate mushrooms for their nutritional benefits and the wide variety of flavors and textures available.

All of this is to say, I totally understand the hesitation when it comes to eating mushrooms, but let me try to change your mind.

In addition to containing nutrients like phosphorous, selenium, copper, potassium, and B vitamins,[45] mushrooms may be a good source of dietary vitamin D.[46] Mushrooms have also been used medicinally throughout history in many cultures around the world, and modern medicine is starting to recognize the benefits of eating these phytochemical-rich fungi, including potential anti-cancer properties.[47]

Mushrooms, when not dried and powdered and sold as smoothie additives, are also really affordable and versatile! They can bring a great meaty texture and unique flavor to a meal, and they are common in many cuisines.

Berries

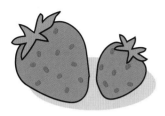

When I talk about berries, I'm not just talking about the ones you can find only in health food stores that are imported from around the world. Yes, goji and açai berries are loaded with vitamins, minerals, and phytonutrients, but so are blackberries, blueberries, cranberries, raspberries, and strawberries! Pretty much all berries are loaded with vitamins, minerals, and a plethora of antioxidant phytonutrients, [48] so pick your favorites and run with it.

On a strict ketogenic diet, it's unlikely that you'll be eating bowlfuls of berries, but working 25 to 50 grams of berries into your carb allowance won't be too difficult. The following list of common berries is presented in order of net carbohydrate content from lowest to highest.

Fresh Berries	Net Carbs per 100g
Raspberries (1¼ cups)	3.2g
Blackberries (scant 1½ cups)	4.9g
Strawberries (1½ cups halved)	6.6g
Ground cherries (scant 1½ cups)	11.2g
Blueberries (1½ cups)	12.5g

Note: Because many superfood berries are only widely available in their dried form, it seemed like an unhelpful comparison to list them here. Dried goji berries, for instance, contain 63.5 grams of net carbs per 100 grams, which equates to 3.7 grams per tablespoon.

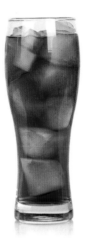

What About Diet Soda?

I'm always hesitant to recommend diet soda because I've heard/read so many accounts of people who have been kicked out of ketosis by drinking it. Other people report that drinking diet soda causes them to start craving sweet foods, which is counterproductive at best and can trigger a binge. If you don't fall into either camp and really need diet soda to function, then go ahead. I just think it's good to be aware of the potential impact.

What About Alcohol?

This is a question I get a *lot*. In short—yes, you can fit alcohol into a ketogenic diet. In fact, many beverage producers now include sugar-free, low-carb, and keto-friendly drinks and mixers in their lineups. The recent popularity jump of hard seltzer is a prime example.

Basically, if you are going to drink alcohol, the lowest-carb options are as follows:

- Hard seltzer
- Unflavored hard alcohol
- Dry wine
- Light beer

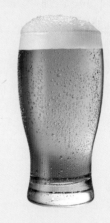

As with anything else, you will want to check the nutrition label (wherever available—most drinks catering to a low-carb crowd provide some form of nutrition information on either the packaging or the manufacturer's website).

In general, unflavored hard alcohol and seltzer are going to be your lowest-carb options, while dry wines and light beers tend to have between 4 and 5 grams of carbs per serving on average.

Saving Money on a Plant-Forward Diet

It's no secret that a nutrient-dense diet made up of high-quality foods can become pricey quickly, but there are a few ways to lower the cost so you can eat well but still stay within budget. I also want to note that these are all things I actually do, and they have definitely helped me bring my grocery costs down!

Keep It Simple

While I enjoy a protein bar or convenience snack from time to time, pretty much everything marketed to keto dieters seems to be insanely expensive. Gluten-free foods have this same issue. I understand that a lot of this is due to the higher cost of ingredients, but it still doesn't mean I want to spend the cash.

When I got started on keto, I didn't really know what I was doing, so I relied pretty heavily on things like shirataki noodles, mock meats, and sugar-free protein bars. While there is nothing wrong with these products, they are on the pricier side, and I found that in the first few weeks of keto I was spending way too much for my budget. Eventually, as I started figuring out what foods I could eat and cooking full meals myself, I began saving lots of money. I still buy all of those items, but I enjoy them in moderation. I also don't rely on them for the majority of my meals, which has saved me loads of money in the long run.

Buy in Bulk

When I talk about bulk buying, I don't mean warehouse stores. Nor am I talking about the bulk aisle in the grocery store (although both of those options can help you save cash). Lots of products become much cheaper when purchased in slightly larger quantities—either online or at those same grocery stores, but in the international foods section or on a lower shelf than the smaller, more expensive containers.

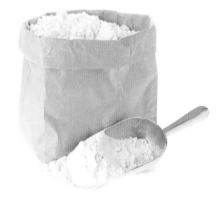

For instance, sesame seeds are often found in the spice section in tiny 2-ounce (56-gram) jars that can cost $5 to $6. But a 1-pound (454-gram) bag of those same seeds costs $4.99 at many online retailers, like Nuts.com. Even crazier, you can often find an 8-ounce (225-gram) bag of sesame seeds for around $3 or $4 in the same grocery aisle as the spices. This is far from the only product that you can buy in bulk in the grocery store, and it drives me crazy.

I usually buy larger packages of ingredients that I use often (various seeds, nutritional yeast, coconut flour, spices) because, while they usually cost more up front, I spend far less overall.

Pass Up (Unnecessary) Supplements

Supplements are a big moneymaker, and the keto diet has not escaped the supplement game by a long shot. In fact, there are whole multilevel marketing schemes dedicated to making you think you *need* to take expensive supplements in order to achieve and/or maintain ketosis. But it's just not true. There is no supplement that you need to take to eat a ketogenic diet—unless your doctor has specifically advised you to take something.

I've said this time and time again, but the only supplements I personally take for keto are electrolytes after workouts (because the body flushes more of them out when in ketosis). That said, you can even replenish electrolytes through eating normal foods and seasoning them with sea salt or pink Himalayan salt. Unrelated to keto, because my diet is entirely plant-based and I burn like crazy in the sun, I take vitamins B_{12} and D,* and I suggest talking to your doctor about those if you're in the same boat.

While your body can produce vitamin D in response to sun exposure, for a good portion of the year most of us are tilted too far away from the sun for this to occur. Additionally, the use of sunscreen can prevent endogenous vitamin D production by blocking UVB rays.

Back to the main point, the following is a quick list of supplements you absolutely do not need to buy. Can they help you get into ketosis faster or give you an energy boost? Sure—I'm not saying they don't "work." I'm just saying they are not necessary and are very expensive.

- Exogenous ketones ("ketone powders")
- Medium-chain triglycerides (often found in oil or powder form)
- Keto coffee, coffee creamers, and beverages in general
- "Keto" protein powder (usually with added MCTs, sometimes with ketones)

Of course, if you have cash to spare and want to try these out, I don't blame you! I've probably tried every type of keto supplement out there, if only to see what the fuss is about. (Fortunately, many are available in single-serving sizes.) While I did notice effects from some of them, and I honestly just enjoy a lot of those keto tea and coffee drinks, most of the time these extras are not in my budget—and I know I'm not alone in that.

Buy Frozen

There is nothing wrong with frozen vegetables and fruit! One of my biggest pet peeves is seeing nutrition professionals eschew the freezer aisle on the grounds that "fresh is best." Yes, fresh, local vegetables are ideal, but frozen produce is usually preserved when it is at its peak and still packs loads of nutrients.

Frozen vegetables are typically much less expensive than their fresh counterparts; some even contain *more* vitamins and minerals,[49] especially if you live in a colder climate (like I do) where many vegetables are trucked in from 3,000 miles away during the winter.

In my kitchen, frozen vegetables and berries are staple items. I pretty much always have some mix of the following on hand:

- Broccoli florets
- Brussels sprouts
- Cauliflower rice and florets
- Mushrooms
- Sliced bell peppers
- Spinach, collards, and kale
- Strawberries, blackberries, and raspberries

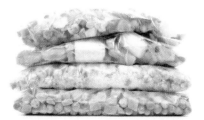

I use these foods in a lot of my recipes and find that keeping them on hand in the freezer is not only cost-effective, but also just really convenient for those nights when I don't have the time or energy to prep a bunch of vegetables for dinner.

I also like to buy some of my favorite vegetables when they're on sale and then prep (wash, stem, peel, chop, etc.) and freeze them for later. I realize that this is a little time-consuming, though, and may not be a possibility for everyone.

What About Canned?

You might be thinking, "What about canned?" Canned vegetables are totally fine as well! They do tend to be slightly overcooked due to the nature of canning, so they usually don't replace their fresh counterparts as well as frozen veggies do. That said, I keep a nice backstock of canned vegetables in my pantry (mostly green beans, spinach, peas, beets, and asparagus), along with dried beans.

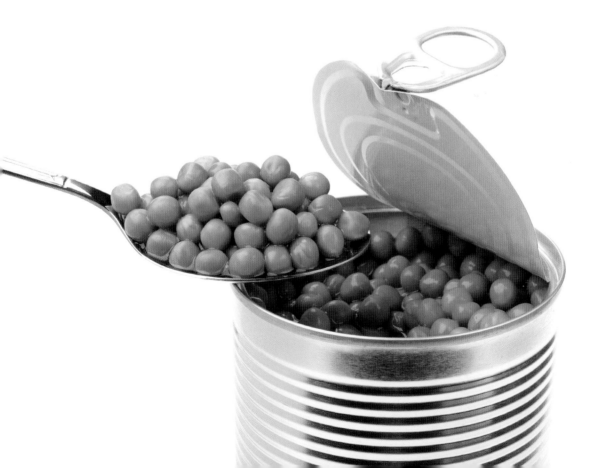

Do Some DIY

Do you *have* to make your own food? No, of course not. However, if you buy sprouts or pretty much anything made with nuts or seeds as the sole ingredient (flour, butter, milk) and you've got a little extra time, I think it's worth the effort to make them. Plus, you then have a use for all those jars you've been hoarding!

Believe it or not, I'm kind of lazy in the kitchen and often prefer to do things the easy way. However, this tendency often conflicts with my frugal side, so there are some things I will buckle down and make myself, especially when the directions say to forget about something on the counter for a while, or when it can be made in less than five minutes.

Sprouts

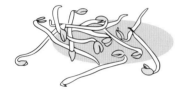

Sprouts are so nutritious, and I like the crunch they add to a dish, but have you looked at the prices? I'm not saying the prices aren't justified for the amount of work and overhead that goes into a commercial growing operation; I'm just saying that for pennies, you can grow the same amount of sprouts on your countertop that would cost $3 to $5 in stores.

Method: You're going to soak seeds or beans and forget about them for a while (sort of). Here's how to sprout: Place 2 tablespoons of seeds or beans in 2 cups (480ml) of water in a sealable container with a ventilated lid. (You can buy sprouting jars at many grocery stores, or you can make your own by securing a piece of mesh over the top of a mason jar with just the rim part of the lid.) Soak for 8 hours. Drain the liquid from the jar through the mesh and set the jar with the seeds aside in a dark place. I store mine upside down so the seeds rest on the screen and water can drip out. Then all you have to do is rinse the sprouts twice daily until they've grown—usually 3 or 4 days. I rinse mine by pouring water through the screen and swirling it around in the jar, then turning the jar upside down to drain. Different sprouts have different directions, so it's worth looking up the specifics for what you want to grow! Once they're "done," keep them in the fridge and use them within a few days.

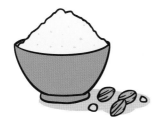

Nut & Seed Flours

Yes, you can buy them, but it's so easy to make your own nut and seed flours that it might be worth adding this task to your meal prepping routine if you have the time.

Method: All you have to do is pulse raw nuts/seeds in a food processor until they are super fine. That's it. Just be sure to stop before you start making nut and seed butters! Which brings me to my next point...

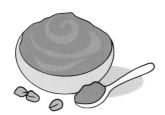

Nut & Seed Butters

Nut and seed butters are also crazy easy to make at home. You just blend nuts or seeds with a bit of oil and salt (or nothing at all) and create your own butter. I find roasting the nuts or seeds first helps release some of the oils so that everything blends together nicely, but you could use raw nuts and seeds as well.

Nut butter blends—my absolute favorite is a combination of dried coconut, cashews, and macadamia nuts—are so much cheaper to make at home than they are to buy that it is worth it to me to spend ten minutes every couple of weeks to do it. Keep in mind that this isn't the case for all nut butters. Almond butter, for example, can be a challenge to make because the nuts are so hard that most home blenders and food processors will not effectively blend them to yield a spreadable nut butter.

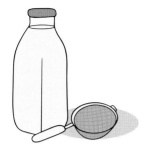

Nut & Seed Milks

Making nut and seed milks is so beyond easy, it's kind of ridiculous. You literally blend any combination of nuts and/or seeds your heart desires with water and then strain out the pulp. That's it. It takes me about 5 minutes total, including straining and pouring the milk into a jar and then cleaning up the milk I spilled on the counter and floor. You can then use the "pulp" as a nut/seed flour in recipes.

Method: I usually start with a 1:3 ratio of nuts/seeds to water and adjust from there, depending on how I'm going to use the milk. This ratio produces a creamy milk that works well in tea or coffee. For a thinner nut milk that is similar to what you find in stores, a 1:5 ratio works well. Soak the nuts/seeds in water that is just off the boil for about a half hour (or in room-temperature water overnight), then drain them and put them in a high-speed blender with more water. Process on high for around a minute, then strain the milk from the solids. The milk is ready to use in recipes or in your morning coffee and can be stored in the fridge for up to 3 days.

If you absolutely despise using a nut milk bag to strain the milk (I really dislike the feeling of squeezing the milk out of the pulp for some reason), I recommend using a fine-mesh sieve instead. You can just press the pulp against the sieve with a spoon, and you don't have to touch it.

Another benefit of making your own nondairy milks is that you can experiment with different combinations. Lately I've been making hazelnut milk for my morning coffee. Also, fun fact: You can make nondairy milk out of different legumes. In addition to making soy milk, I've experimented with chickpeas and peas with varying degrees of success.

Making your own nut and seed products may seem like a lot of work, but in reality, you could make nut/seed flour, butter, and milk for the week in less than 30 minutes while also doing some other kitchen prep.

Notes on Ethical Sourcing

I said I wasn't going to get preachy, but I want to mention a few things on sourcing certain foods. Part of the reason I stick with a vegan diet is to limit the amount of harm I do to animals, the planet, and my fellow humans. Usually, when the media discusses a cruelty-free diet, the first of those three categories takes precedent, and the environment and humanity are given less consideration (though this focus is changing).

In fact, when I was trying to find resources for cruelty-free products, most of what came up was animal related. Don't get me wrong, I love animals, and I don't want my lifestyle to contribute to their suffering, but I feel that way about people and the planet, too. I'm not going to go into the details of why each of the following foods poses ethical concerns, but I highly recommend checking out a study by Ainhoa Magrach and María José Sanz, called "Environmental and Social Consequences of the Increase in the Demand for 'Superfoods' World-Wide," which can be found at https://doi.org/10.1002/pan3.10085.

The following list of foods can pose ethical challenges because their cultivation and distribution rely on either exploitative or environmentally unsustainable practices—and often both are at play:

- All animal products (meat, fish, eggs, and dairy)
- Almonds
- Avocados
- Cacao
- Cashews
- Coconuts
- Coffee
- Hearts of palm
- Palm oil

(Of course, many other foods also pose ethical challenges, but since they are not mentioned in this book, nor are they typically part of a ketogenic diet, it seems unnecessary to discuss them in this context.)

This whole section isn't to say you shouldn't eat these foods. We all have different priorities, and ethical sourcing might not be yours at the moment. So feel free to skip over this part! If ethical sourcing is a priority for you, there are companies that go to great lengths to ensure that their business model does not negatively impact their workers or the economy and environment of their growing region.

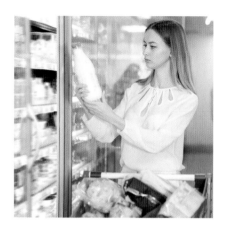

That said, finding ethical sources can be challenging, especially since most brands do not openly disclose their sourcing. This is one of the things that drew me to Thrive Market (no, this is not an ad). They list information about sourcing for many of their products and for all of their private-label items. Additionally, they make a concerted effort to procure ingredients for their private label as ethically as possible and carry other brands that do the same.

Most of the time, when a brand works hard to source a product ethically, they are excited about it and eager to share that information. So, a quick way to determine whether a company has made an effort to be as ethical and sustainable as possible is to check for any combination of the following labels (usually accompanied by a seal) on the packaging:

- **Bird Friendly (Smithsonian):** Found on bags of coffee, this label indicates that the coffee beans were grown and harvested in ways that protect the forests and birds in the area surrounding the farms.
- **Certified B Corporation:** This label is given to companies that adhere to rigorous criteria in terms of how their practices impact workers, customers, and the community as well as the environment.
- **Certified Humane:** For those who consume animal products, a Certified Humane seal indicates that the animals were raised and slaughtered in the most humane way possible.
- **Equal Exchange:** Equal Exchange is a worker-owned, democratic co-op of Fair Trade Certified chocolate, coffee, and tea growers.

- **Fair for Life:** Fair for Life certifies not only products but also raw materials throughout the supply chain to work toward completely sustainably and ethically produced goods.
- **Fair Trade Certified:** A certification for all types of food and consumer products requiring stringent standards for workers' rights, fair labor practices, and responsible land management.
- **Forest Stewardship Council (FSC):** Formed as a response to rampant global deforestation, the council certifies that manufacturers' materials are from sustainably managed forests. You'll see the FSC logo on a lot of food packaging.
- **Leaping Bunny:** This logo is found on cruelty-free (free of animal testing at all stages) cosmetics, body care products, cleaning products, and animal care products.
- **Rainforest Alliance:** This organization partners with farmers and forest communities to promote sustainable land practices and with local governments to enact environmentally beneficial policies. You can find its seal on many products grown in rainforests, including bananas, cacao, coffee, tea, and even flowers.
- **Roundtable on Sustainable Palm Oil (RSPO):** This seal is given to products made with sustainable palm oil that also meet high standards for ethical labor and environmental practices.

These labels aren't all perfect, but they're a start, and certainly better than nothing. There are also plenty of other organizations across all sectors of the consumer market (not just agriculture) that have their own labels.

I'm not trying to guilt anyone or judge people's food choices, but rather aiming to provide a little information. I'm also not saying *I* am perfect. I only found out about a lot of the impact of these products within the past few years, and I am aware that I probably consume a ton of other products that have a detrimental effect—but I'm trying!

And yes, sourcing foods (and everything else) in an ethical manner is far more expensive than buying conventionally produced food, but this is something I am willing to pay more for, or to do without.

The following websites can help you find brands that align with your own beliefs and provide more information on certification requirements:

- **Certified B Corporation (bcorporation.net):** Information about the criteria for becoming a certified B Corp along with lists of companies that have received the certification.

- **Certified Humane (certifiedhumane.org):** Includes the full humane standards for each species, as well as lists of certified producers. There is also a "where to buy" tool to help locate Certified Humane products.

- **End Slavery Now (endslaverynow.org):** Provides educational resources about the forms of slavery that exist in many supply chains along with shopping guides to help you avoid companies that rely on slave labor.

- **Environmental Working Group (ewg.org):** Provides information on health and the environment, including a rundown of pesticide residues found on vegetables and fruits, ingredient breakdowns of cosmetics, and a tool to search and identify contaminants in local drinking water.

- **Ethical Consumer (ethicalconsumer.org):** Provides information on purchasing ethically produced consumer items across all sectors.

- **Leaping Bunny Program (leapingbunny.org):** Lists cruelty-free companies on the site and offers an app to search for cruelty-free products while shopping.

- **Rainforest Alliance (rainforest-alliance.org):** A tool for helping to create a world that is more in harmony with nature through lifestyle choices by providing information along with actionable steps that go beyond just purchasing the products it certifies.

- **Slave Free Chocolate (slavefreechocolate.org):** Lists chocolate producers (an industry that heavily relies on child labor, often slave labor) that not only engage in ethical labor practices but also work to end unethical practices in the industry.

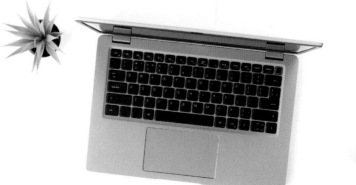

How to Use These Recipes

Experiment!

I firmly believe that a recipe is meant to be a guideline and is open for customization (baking less so, but you get the point). Once you've got the main idea of the dish down, you can experiment by adding, substituting, or eliminating certain ingredients. You'll notice that many of the recipes have variations that offer different flavor profiles: this is because I get bored easily and love experimenting with food and flavors. I highly encourage you to do the same thing!

Keep in mind that the recipes in this book are written with flexibility in mind, whether it's the flavorings, the vegetables, or the protein. So, while many of the entrée recipes list a recommended protein, don't let that recommendation limit you. Really, if you absolutely hate tofu, you don't need to use the tofu-based protein!

You can also add proteins (see pages 170 to 201) to all of the salads and soups to make them a full meal. See the Meal Pairings on pages 90 and 91 for lots of ideas for mixing and matching.

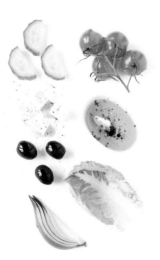

Choose Your Own Adventure!

When I was in elementary school, *Choose Your Own Adventure* books were really popular. If you've never read one, the concept is pretty simple—you read a story that progresses to a certain fork in the road, and then you choose from (usually two) options where you want the plot to progress. This continues a few more times until you arrive at the conclusion.

What was cool about these books is that you could reread the story a few times and make different decisions, and the outcome could be completely different. It was exciting to see how each option turned out. This is how the recipes in this book are designed.

Take a Food Vacation

One of my favorite ways to explore new flavors is to take what I call a food vacation: I pick a random location (EarthRoulette. com is my favorite website for this) and then do a deep dive into the food culture of that area. There are so many region- and culture-specific cookbooks out there as well as creators online who love to share their regional dishes. You can learn so much about the history and overall culture of an

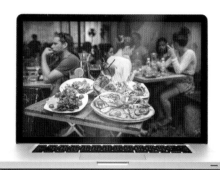

area just by digging into its cuisine and commonly used ingredients. After a solid amount of reading and watching, I'll pick a bunch of recipes to make and some seasoning blends to try over the course of a week. Eventually, many of those seasonings and dishes make their way into my regular meal rotation.

Food Allergy/Sensitivity Concerns & Making Substitutions

As someone who has spent years substituting ingredients in recipes to accommodate food allergies and dietary preferences, I know how annoying it can be to buy a cookbook and then struggle to find recipes to make from it. With this in mind, I've tried to create recipes that are relatively allergy-friendly, aiming to keep the most common allergens to a minimum or at least to provide substitutions for them.

I've listed common substitutions within recipe notes, but I wanted to point out the most common ones here:

- **Hemp seeds** can be replaced with shelled sunflower seeds or pumpkin seeds (pepitas) in many recipes, with the exception of the Hemp Seed Tabbouleh (page 134).
- **Almond flour** can be replaced with sunflower seed flour.

- **Lupin flour** can be replaced with soy flour or chickpea flour.
- **Soy-based tofu and tempeh** can be replaced with soy-free versions of these proteins (like hempeh or pumpkin seed tofu) or with soy-free mock meats.
- **Mock meats** can be replaced with tofu, tempeh, or seitan for a less-processed protein.

In addition:

- **Ground flaxseed and ground chia seed** can be used interchangeably.
- **Almond butter, peanut butter, and sunflower seed butter** are all interchangeable.

If you are tracking, just keep in mind that the nutrition profiles of these ingredients do vary.

A Note on Listed Allergens

All of the recipes in this book are gluten- and grain-free; except for the protein toppers on pages 184 to 201, they are also free from animal products like fish,

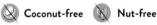 Coconut-free  Nut-free Peanut-free  Soy-free

shellfish, eggs, and dairy. The allergen icons at the tops of the recipes are based on the first ingredient choice listed and do not take into account any suggested accompaniments or garnishes. (Same goes for the nutrition info.) In many cases, you can use the second option to make the recipe coconut-free, nut-free, peanut-free, or soy-free to meet your dietary needs.

Protein Toppers & Meal Pairings

While some of the entrée recipes already contain a protein—Shepherd's Pie (page 158), for example—many need a protein boost to make them more filling and protein-rich. That's where the protein toppers come in! At the end of the Entrée chapter, starting on page 170, there is a section of protein recipes that can be added to the main dishes to make a complete meal. You could also add them to the salads for the same effect, or even pick a few sides to combine with them. There are so many possibilities!

Why structure things this way? One of the most challenging parts of keto is how rigid it can be, and I wanted to provide you with a little flexibility.

I often receive messages from people saying that they have to make two full meals because their spouse eats meat, or they're trying to cut down on eating meat but really don't like tofu and struggle to find other options. The protein section should help with that! Since I don't eat or cook meat (I don't even know how!), I enlisted the help of the awesome recipe developer Launie Kettler from TeenyTinyKitchen. com for the recipes on pages 184 to 201. She created eight fantastic animal protein toppers to pair with the completely plant-based recipes in the rest of the book so your whole family can eat the same meal without too much hassle.

My husband isn't vegan, so usually I make us one main dish (like the Moroccan-Inspired Butternut Squash Stew on page 142) and cook a protein for myself (usually the Cumin Spice "Meatballs" variation on page 178) while he cooks his own protein (or just eats mine). Sometimes I make this same main dish with Super Crispy Baked Tofu (page 172) on top instead for a different texture, and sometimes I just top it with some Vegan Feta (page 180) that I have stored in the fridge. It's all about ease!

If you don't want to think too much when trying to put together low-carb meal pairings (especially if you're fairly new to low-carb or ketogenic diets), I've created these favorite pairings of entrées, proteins, and sides as a starting point:

- Moroccan-Inspired Butternut Squash Stew (page 142) + Cumin Spice "Meatballs" (page 178) + Harissa Roasted Carrots (page 218) and/or Ras el Hanout Mashed Butternut Squash (page 230)
- Falafel Waffles (page 98) + Yogurt Dill Sauce (page 240) + Rainbow Veggie Pilaf (page 214)
- Garlic-Chive Super Crispy Baked Tofu (page 172) + Sesame-Garlic Kale (page 212) + Sea Vegetable Salad (page 204)
- Empanada-Inspired Collard Wraps (page 150) + Chimichurri (page 242) + Chimichurri Roasted Celeriac (page 222)
- Balsamic-Marinated Skillet Tempeh (page 176) + Balsamic Beets & Greens (page 216)
- Lemon Pepper Baked Tofu OR Mediterranean Baked Tofu (page 170) + Ratatouille (page 226)

- Sauerkraut Soup (page 122) + Tempeh Bacon (page 174)
- Fauxtato Leek Soup (page 124) + Tempeh Bacon (page 174)
- Mushroom Stroganoff (page 146) + Mushroom "Meatballs" (page 178) OR Tempeh Bacon (page 174)

Measuring Ingredients

All of the recipes in this book include both imperial volume measurements and their metric weight or volume equivalents for measurements of ¼ cup or greater.

While I often use a kitchen scale to measure ingredients, when I'm using volume measurements (like cups or tablespoons) for dry ingredients, I scoop the ingredient out of the container and then scrape off the excess with the back of a knife. So, unless specifically stated, measurements are not "rounded" or "heaping" cups or tablespoons. This is particularly important for keto baking, as many ingredients (such as coconut flour) do not act like traditional baking ingredients and need to be measured precisely.

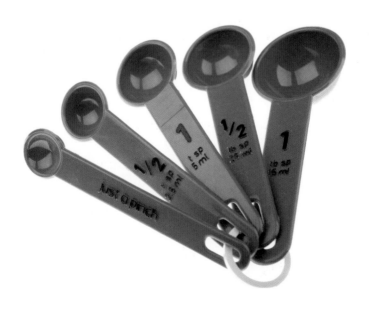

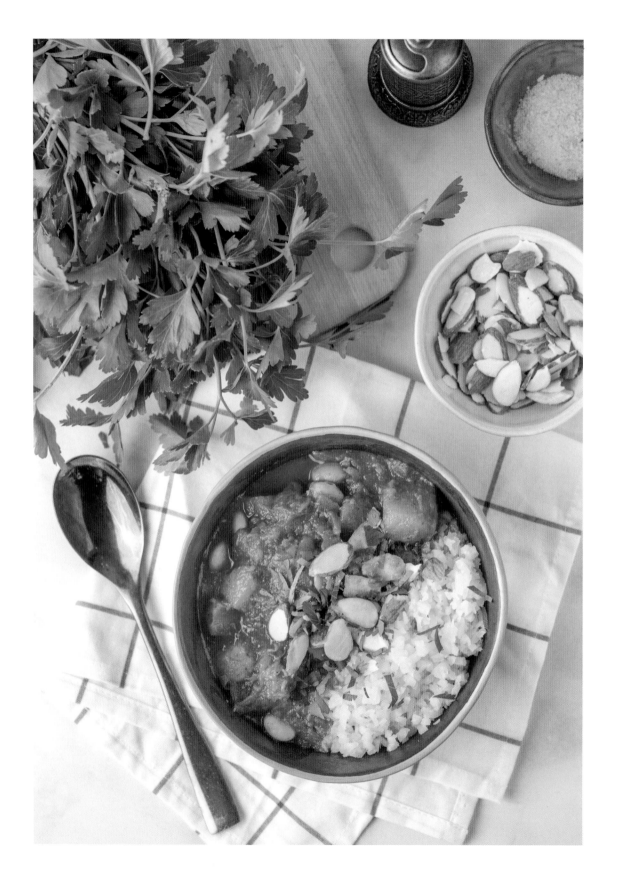

Recipes

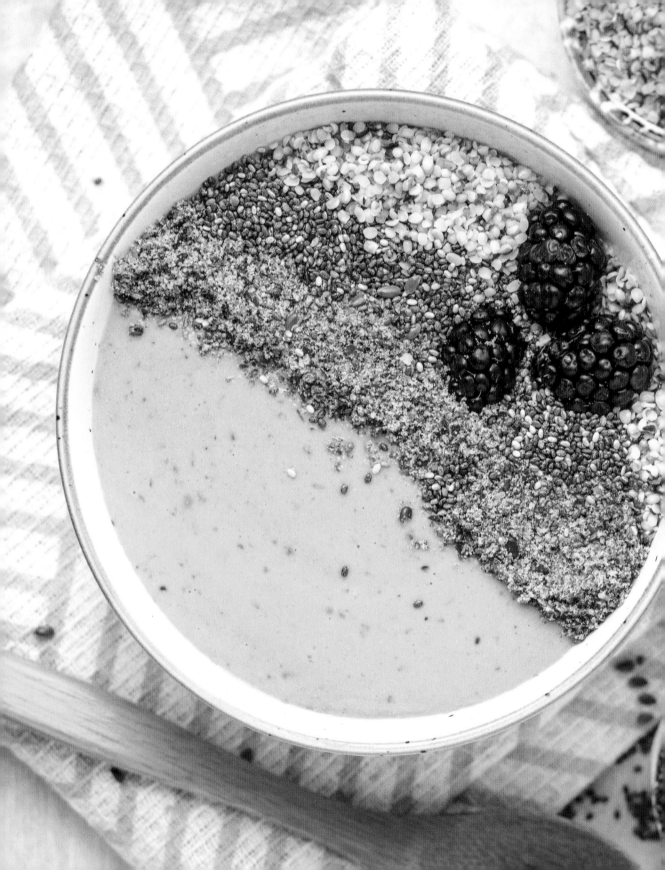

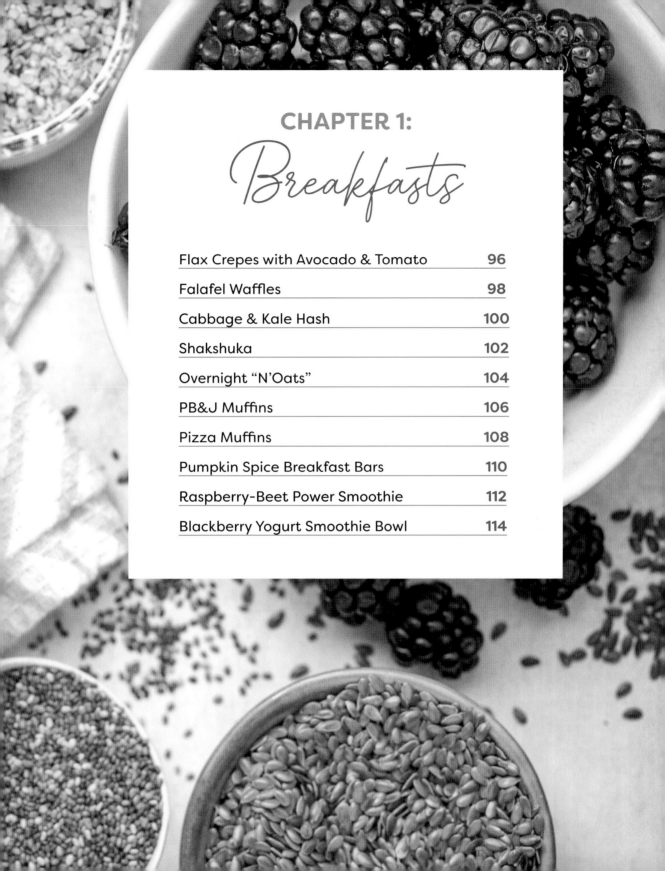

CHAPTER 1:

Breakfasts

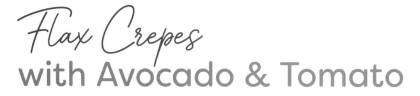

Flax Crepes with Avocado & Tomato

YIELD: 3 crepes (1 per serving)
PREP TIME: 10 minutes
COOK TIME: 8 minutes

Are these crepes? Are they tortillas? I don't really know what to call them. I know they're not pancakes or wraps, and they're not blintzes, either. I guess they're kind of a flatbread? A really, really flat bread.

No matter what they're called, they're easy to make and store well. I like to make a few batches at a time and keep them in the fridge for when I want a quick meal during the week. This avocado and tomato combo is my favorite, especially in the summer with an heirloom tomato. Yes, please. For a protein boost, I sometimes add a few slices of Tempeh Bacon (page 174).

CREPES

1 cup (240ml) hot water

1 cup (112g) ground flaxseed

1 teaspoon granulated garlic

½ teaspoon salt

¼ teaspoon ground black pepper

FILLING

1 medium Hass avocado (about 7½ ounces/212g), halved and pitted

1 large Roma tomato (about 3½ ounces/100g)

Salt and ground black pepper

TO STORE: Refrigerate the crepes separately from the avocado and tomato in tightly sealed containers for up to 3 days. The leftovers are best eaten cold.

- **To make the crepes:** In a bowl, whisk together all of the crepe ingredients. Let sit for about 5 minutes, until the batter thickens to the consistency of thin pancake batter.

- Heat a medium nonstick frying pan over medium-low heat. To cook each crepe, scoop ¼ cup (60ml) of batter into the center of the pan. It will start bubbling and spread out into a round that is about 6 inches (15cm) in diameter. Cook for about 2 minutes, until the bubbling stops and the top is no longer tacky to the touch. Flip the crepe and cook for another 30 seconds on the other side, until golden.

- Repeat with the remaining batter to make three crepes.

- **To fill the crepes:** Scoop the avocado flesh into a small bowl and mash with a fork. Divide into three portions and spread over half of each crepe. Slice the tomato and distribute the slices evenly among the crepes, placing the slices over the mashed avocado. Season with salt and pepper to taste and fold the crepes in half to enjoy.

NUTRITION:
285 calories | **22.8g** fat | **8.2g** protein | **16.9g** total carbs | **3.1g** net carbs

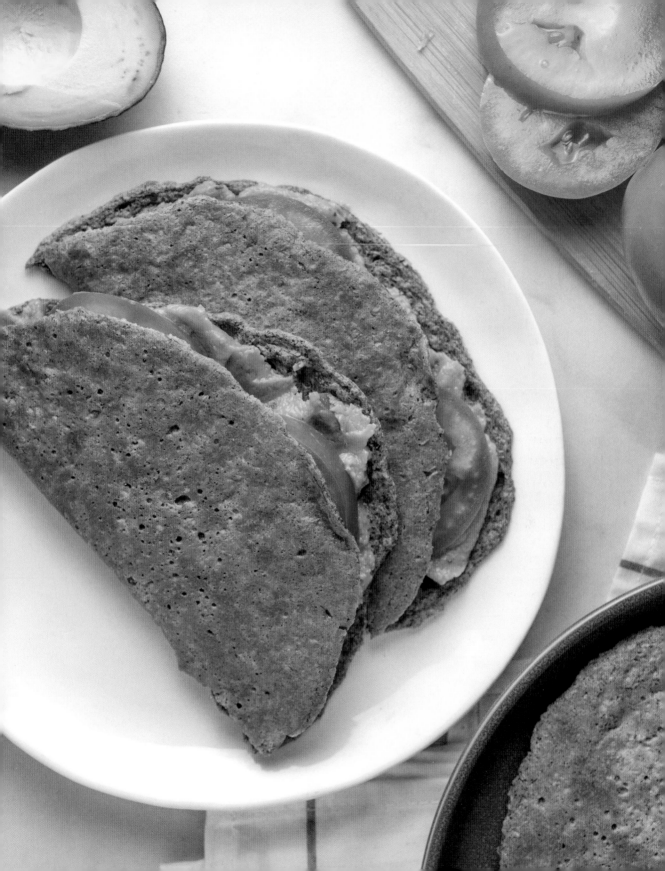

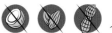

Falafel Waffles

YIELD: 2 waffles (1 per serving)

PREP TIME: 10 minutes

COOK TIME: 10 minutes

Have I mentioned my love of falafel yet? Truly, falafel is one of my all-time favorite foods, my green eggs and ham. I could eat it forever and be happy. Because of my deep and abiding love for this delicious chickpea-based food, I have made loads of keto-friendly variations over the years. These falafel waffles (I really want to call them *fal-affles*) are my latest fixation.

Instead of making falafel waffles with chickpeas, I opt for lupin flour, which has keto-friendly macros. You could also use an equal measure of soy flour, almond flour, or sunflower seed flour. I have made them with unflavored protein powder, too, and they came out surprisingly tasty, though a bit protein-powdery and not my first choice.

½ cup (60g) lupin flour

⅓ cup (50g) frozen chopped spinach, thawed

¼ cup (16g) nutritional yeast

1 tablespoon psyllium husks

1 tablespoon dried parsley

1½ teaspoons ground cumin

1 teaspoon dehydrated onion flakes

½ teaspoon granulated garlic

¼ teaspoon ground black pepper

½ cup (120ml) water

2 tablespoons tahini

1 tablespoon extra-virgin olive oil, plus extra for the waffle iron

SUGGESTED ACCOMPANIMENTS

Chopped fresh parsley

Yogurt Dill Sauce (page 240)

Tahini

- In a medium bowl, stir together the lupin flour, spinach, nutritional yeast, psyllium husks, parsley, cumin, onion flakes, granulated garlic, and pepper until well combined.

- Add the water, tahini, and oil and stir until the batter is smooth. Let sit for 3 to 5 minutes, until the psyllium has gelled and the batter has become quite thick. Divide the batter into two equal portions.

- Preheat a waffle iron according to the manufacturer's instructions. Once it's warmed up a bit, grease the iron with olive oil so the waffles don't stick.

- Place half of the batter in the center of the waffle iron. Cook for about 5 minutes, until golden brown.

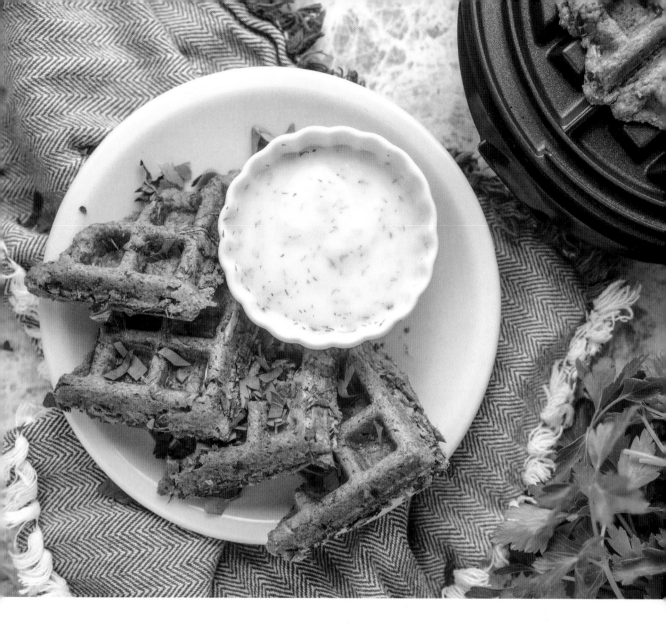

TO STORE: Refrigerate in an airtight container for up to 3 days.

TO REHEAT: Warm in a preheated 300°F (150°C) oven for 5 minutes, until heated through.

- Carefully remove the waffle from the waffle iron. To make this task easier, I like to (carefully) shimmy a chopstick under the waffle to loosen it a little, then free it using two forks or chopsticks for support.

- Regrease the waffle iron and repeat with the remaining batter.

- Garnish with fresh parsley and serve with a drizzle of yogurt sauce and/or tahini, if desired.

NUTRITION:
282 calories | **17.6g** fat | **19.5g** protein | **23.4g** total carbs | **6.4g** net carbs

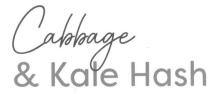

Cabbage & Kale Hash

YIELD: 4 servings

PREP TIME: 15 minutes

COOK TIME: 16 minutes

Looking at the ingredients for this recipe, I can imagine you thinking that I'm taking a lot of liberties with the word *hash,* which...yes, yes I am. Instead of meat and potatoes and maybe some vegetables, we have tempeh and cauliflower and loads more vegetables.

I usually make this hash without any sort of protein and serve it alongside a tofu scramble or with mock sausage for myself and then make scrambled eggs for my husband. When I only feel like making one big meal, though, I crumble tempeh directly into the pan (see the variation below).

2 tablespoons extra-virgin olive oil

½ medium yellow, orange, or red bell pepper (about 2 ounces/60g), cored, seeded, and chopped

1 teaspoon dried thyme leaves

½ teaspoon salt

¼ teaspoon ground black pepper

2 teaspoons minced garlic

2 cups (175g) chopped green cabbage

1 cup (100g) chopped cauliflower florets

1 cup (85g) chopped kale

1½ teaspoons apple cider vinegar (optional)

Chopped fresh parsley, for garnish (optional)

- Heat the oil in a large frying pan over medium-low heat. Add the bell pepper, thyme, salt, and black pepper and cook for about 5 minutes, until the pepper softens. Add the garlic and continue to cook for another minute.

- Add the cabbage, cauliflower, kale, and vinegar and stir everything together. Cover the pan and cook for another 10 minutes, until all of the vegetables are soft. Transfer to a serving bowl and garnish with parsley, if desired.

TO STORE: Refrigerate in an airtight container for up to 3 days.

TO REHEAT: Warm in a small frying pan over low heat for about 5 minutes, until the desired temperature is reached.

VARIATION: Tempeh Hash. Crumble an 8-ounce (225-g) package of tempeh and cook it with the bell pepper and seasonings so it is well incorporated with the vegetables.

NUTRITION:
93 calories | **7.3g** fat | **2g** protein | **6.7g** total carbs | **3.7g** net carbs

NUTRITION (Tempeh Hash):
200 calories | **12g** fat | **12.1g** protein | **12.4g** total carbs | **4.9g** net carbs

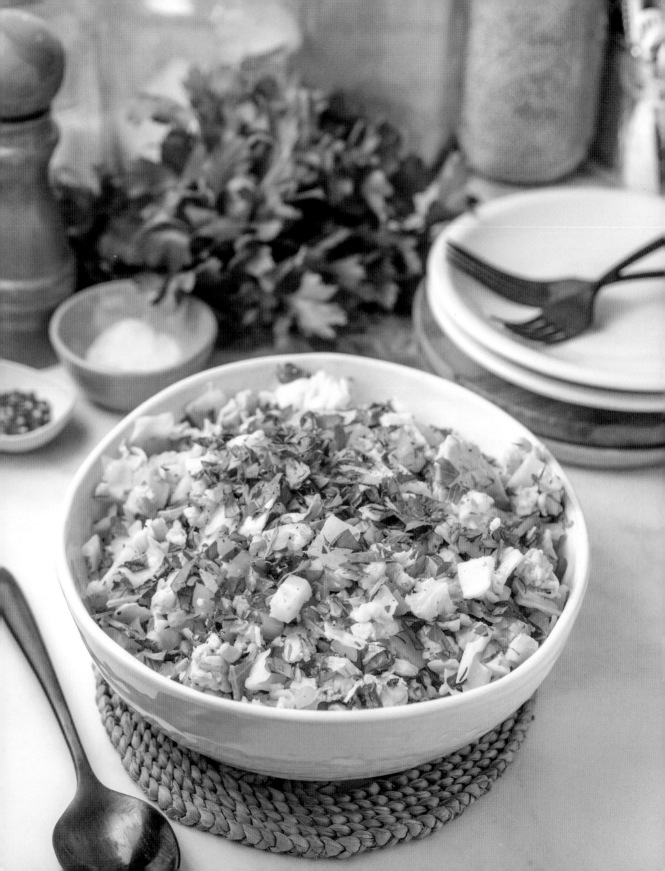

Shakshuka

YIELD: 3 servings

PREP TIME: 10 minutes (not including time to make egg cups)

COOK TIME: 21 minutes, plus time to cook eggs (if using)

If you aren't familiar with this spicy tomato dish, you are missing out! Shakshuka originated somewhere in North Africa in the mid-sixteenth century. As with many classic dishes, the exact origin is oft-disputed, and there are many regional variations. Like any recipe that is converted to be both vegan and keto-friendly, this isn't a traditional shakshuka, but rather an adaptation.

I offer a totally plant-based version, but with an egg substitute option, as I always make shakshuka with eggs for my husband, who doesn't tolerate any beans. You could also make this dish with a vegan egg replacer like Just Egg in place of the egg cups.

If you are making the Lupin "Egg" Cups, I recommend putting them in the oven before starting the shakshuka so that everything finishes at roughly the same time.

2 tablespoons extra-virgin olive oil

½ small onion (about 1¼ ounces/35g), chopped

½ small yellow, orange, or red bell pepper (about 1¼ ounces/35g), cored, seeded, and chopped

¼ teaspoon salt

2 teaspoons minced garlic

2 teaspoons smoked paprika

1 teaspoon ground cumin

½ (14½-ounce/411g) can diced tomatoes with juice

1 medium zucchini (about 7 ounces/200g), grated

1 recipe Lupin "Egg" Cups (page 182), or 6 medium eggs

Ground black pepper, for garnish

Chopped fresh parsley, for garnish

- Heat the oil in a medium frying pan over medium-low heat. Add the onion, bell pepper, and salt and cook, stirring occasionally, until soft, about 5 minutes.

- Add the garlic, paprika, and cumin and cook for another minute. Add the tomatoes and zucchini and stir to combine. Cover the pan and let simmer for 15 minutes, until the vegetables have softened, stirring in a little water if the excess liquid evaporates.

- **If serving with egg cups,** divide the vegetable mixture among three bowls and top with two egg cups each, then garnish with black pepper and parsley.

- **If serving with eggs,** make six wells in the vegetable mixture and crack an egg into each (I recommend cracking each egg into a small bowl first to prevent any shell pieces from falling into the pan). Return the lid to the pan and simmer until the eggs are cooked to your liking. Garnish with black pepper and parsley and serve.

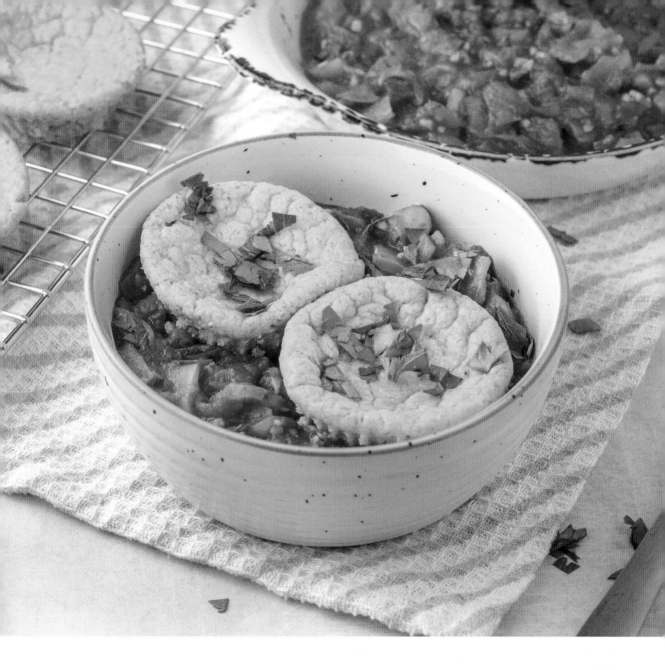

TO STORE: Refrigerate the vegetables and egg cups separately in sealed containers for up to 3 days. Enjoy cold or reheat.

TO REHEAT: Warm the vegetables in a small frying pan over low heat for about 5 minutes, until the desired temperature is reached.

NUTRITION (with Lupin "Egg" Cups):
291 calories | **21g** fat | **11.8g** protein | **19.7g** total carbs | **11g** net carbs

NUTRITION (with eggs):
266 calories | **19.1g** fat | **13.7g** protein | **11.4g** total carbs | **8.4g** net carbs

Overnight "N'Oats"

YIELD: 1 serving

PREP TIME: 5 minutes, plus at least 15 minutes to chill

Overnight oats are one of those food trends that are just so appealing to me. Toss a bunch of ingredients in a jar, leave it in the fridge, and wake up to a breakfast that is ready to go—what could be better? Of course, oats are pretty high in carbohydrates, so when I'm eating keto or low-carb, I make "not oats" instead.

While these don't really need the whole night to set up, I find it convenient to mix up a batch while I'm already in the kitchen making dinner and stick the jar in the fridge for the next day.

2 tablespoons hulled hemp seeds (see Notes)

2 tablespoons ground flaxseed (see Notes)

2 tablespoons vanilla protein powder

2 tablespoons coconut flour

¾ cup (180ml) nondairy milk of choice

TO STORE: Refrigerate in the sealed jar for up to 2 days.

NOTES: This base recipe is really adaptable. If you don't have hemp seeds, you can use an equivalent measure of any nut or seed flour. You can also substitute an equal measure of chia seeds for the ground flaxseed. And while I often just make the base recipe, I love experimenting and trying out new flavor combinations. I encourage you to play around with the variations listed here and come up with your own as well!

Place all of the ingredients in an 8-ounce (240-ml) lidded jar and stir to combine. Secure the lid and refrigerate for at least 15 minutes or overnight to thicken.

VARIATIONS:

Maple-Pecan N'Oats. Reduce the amount of nondairy milk to ½ cup plus 2 tablespoons (150ml) and add 2 tablespoons sugar-free maple syrup and 2 tablespoons chopped pecans.

Mocha N'Oats. Use chocolate protein powder instead of vanilla and add 1 teaspoon instant espresso and 1 tablespoon cacao nibs or unsweetened chocolate chips.

Coconut-Lime N'Oats. Use coconut milk as the nondairy milk and add 2 tablespoons unsweetened coconut flakes and the grated zest and juice of ½ lime.

Lavender-"Honey" N'Oats. Add a pinch of ground dried lavender and 1 tablespoon sugar-free mock honey (such as Harmless Hunny).

Apple-Cinnamon N'Oats (medium-carb). Add ¼ cup (60ml) unsweetened applesauce and ¼ teaspoon ground cinnamon.

NUTRITION (BASE RECIPE):
301 calories | **18.7g** fat | **21.2g** protein | **15.2g** total carbs | **4.2g** net carbs

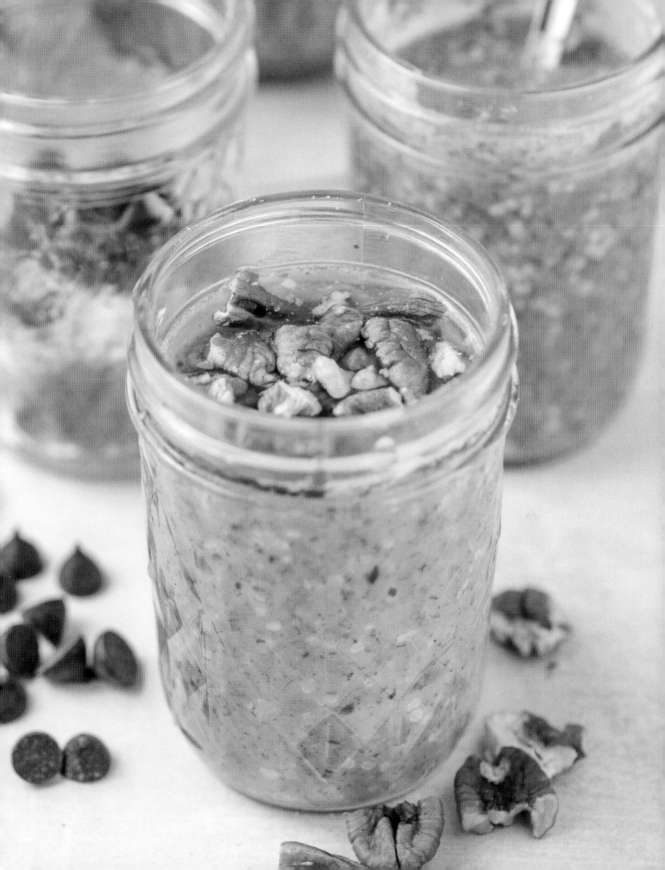

PB&J Muffins

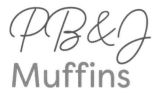

YIELD: 5 muffins (1 per serving)

PREP TIME: 15 minutes

COOK TIME: 35 minutes

I always have freeze-dried berries on hand for baking. I like using them for several reasons. First, they keep for a super long time and retain their flavor well, and unlike frozen berries, there's no freezer burn to worry about! Because they are freeze-dried, I also don't have to worry about extra liquid in the batter or weird temperature differences that occur when using frozen berries. And they suspend in batter really well instead of sinking to the bottom.

If you can't find freeze-dried berries, swirling a teaspoon of sugar-free jam into each muffin portion before baking will work as well!

¼ cup plus 2 tablespoons (96g) unsweetened peanut butter

2 tablespoons softened coconut oil

½ cup (120ml) warm water (see Note)

2 tablespoons ground flaxseed

2 tablespoons granulated sweetener (see page 69)

1 teaspoon vanilla extract

1 teaspoon apple cider vinegar

½ cup (5g) freeze-dried strawberries, plus extra for garnish

¼ cup (28g) coconut flour

½ teaspoon baking powder

¼ teaspoon baking soda

- Preheat the oven to 350°F (177°C) and line five wells of a standard-size muffin pan with paper liners, or have a silicone muffin pan on hand.

- In a medium bowl, mash together the peanut butter and coconut oil. This doesn't have to be perfect, because the warm water will help to mix everything better. Stir in the warm water, ground flaxseed, sweetener, vanilla, and vinegar and keep mixing until everything is fully combined. Let sit for about 5 minutes so the flax has time to gel up.

- In a separate small bowl, fork-whisk the strawberries, coconut flour, baking powder, and baking soda.

- Carefully stir the dry ingredients into the wet just until combined. Let the batter sit for 3 minutes so the coconut flour absorbs some of the liquid and the baking soda reacts to give the batter its first bit of lift.

- Distribute the batter evenly among the muffin cups, filling each about three-quarters full and making sure to smooth over any large peaks. Bake for 30 to 35 minutes, until the tops are firm and the muffins are golden around the edges. Remove from the oven and let cool and set up in the pan for about 10 minutes before removing.

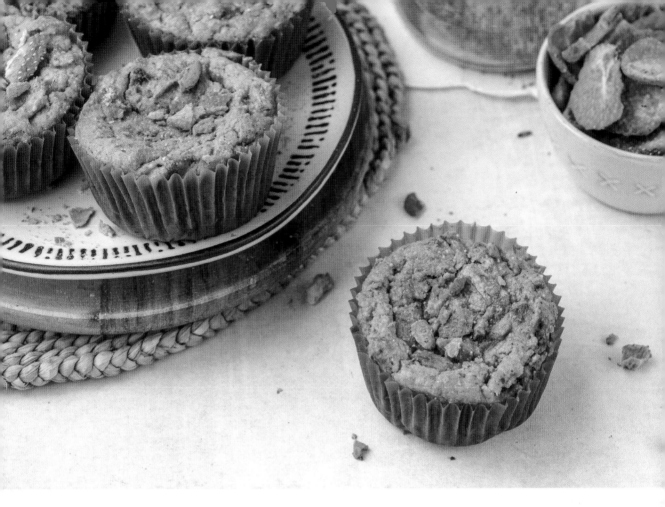

TO STORE: Store in a lidded container at room temperature for up to 3 days or in the refrigerator for up to 5 days.

NOTE: The water should not feel hot to the touch; otherwise, it will prematurely activate the baking powder and the muffins will not rise. The water should just be warm enough that it doesn't cause the coconut oil to harden.

• For extra color (and flavor), crumble a piece of freeze-dried strawberry over the top of each muffin.

VARIATIONS:

Chocolate–Peanut Butter Muffins. Replace the freeze-dried strawberries with 2 tablespoons unsweetened chocolate chips.

Crunchy Peanut Butter Muffins. Replace the freeze-dried strawberries with 2 tablespoons chopped peanuts.

NUTRITION:
205 calories | **16.9g** fat | **6g** protein | **13.7g** total carbs | **4.7g** sugar alcohols | **4g** net carbs

NUTRITION (Chocolate–Peanut Butter Muffins):
230 calories | **19.6g** fat | **6.7g** protein | **16.4g** total carbs | **4.7g** sugar alcohols | **3.5g** net carbs

NUTRITION (Crunchy Peanut Butter Muffins):
218 calories | **18.3g** fat | **6.7g** protein | **13.4g** total carbs | **4.7g** sugar alcohols | **3.7g** net carbs

Pizza Muffins

YIELD: 4 muffins (1 per serving)
PREP TIME: 10 minutes
COOK TIME: 25 minutes

I'm a big fan of savory breakfasts, and these pizza muffins have long been a staple in my household. I typically make a batch for myself and then an egg-based batch for my husband for breakfasts on the weekend (neither one of us is a weekday breakfast person). If you want to make more than four muffins, the recipe doubles really well.

I typically have a couple of these for breakfast with some Cabbage & Kale Hash (page 100) on the side. Sometimes I split them in half and make tiny sandwiches with some Tempeh Bacon (page 174) in the middle. They're surprisingly versatile!

My favorite type of dairy-free cheese for topping these muffins is the shredded mozzarella from Violife, but pretty much any nondairy (or dairy!) shreds will taste good.

½ cup (120ml) low-sugar tomato sauce

¼ cup (16g) nutritional yeast

2 tablespoons tahini

2 tablespoons water

1 tablespoon extra-virgin olive oil

¼ cup (30g) lupin flour

2 tablespoons coconut flour

1 teaspoon baking powder

1 teaspoon psyllium husks

½ teaspoon dried oregano leaves

¼ teaspoon salt

2 tablespoons shredded dairy-free or regular cheese, for topping (optional)

Red pepper flakes, for garnish (optional)

- Preheat the oven to 375°F (190°C) and line four wells of a standard-size muffin pan with paper liners, or have a silicone muffin pan on hand.

- In a medium bowl, stir together the tomato sauce, nutritional yeast, tahini, water, and oil until smooth.

- In a separate small bowl, whisk together the lupin flour, coconut flour, baking powder, psyllium husks, oregano, and salt until thoroughly combined.

- Fold the dry ingredients into the wet and continue to stir until no clumps remain. Let the batter sit for about 5 minutes so the psyllium starts to gel and the coconut flour absorbs the liquid.

- Divide the batter evenly among the four muffin cups, filling each almost to the top. Smooth over any peaks with your finger so they don't burn. Bake for 25 minutes, or until the muffins are firm to the touch and golden around the edges. If you want to top them with cheese, place 1½ teaspoons of shredded cheese on top of each muffin after 15 minutes of baking.

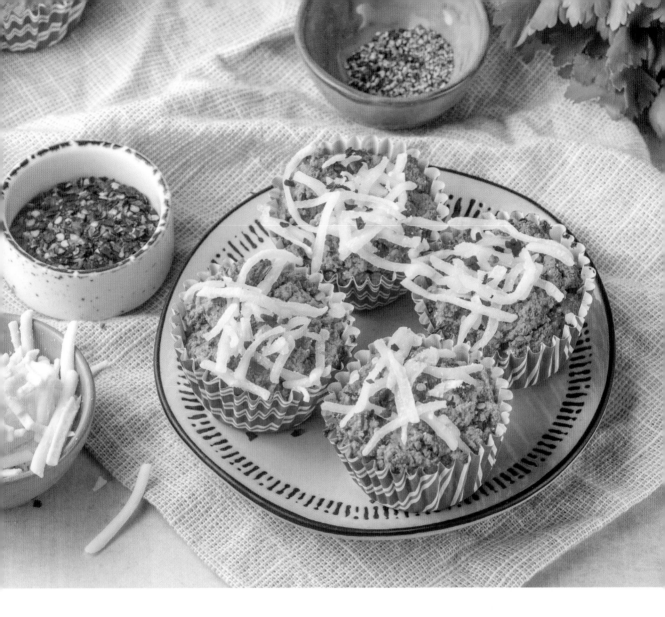

TO STORE: Refrigerate in an airtight container for up to 3 days.

TO REHEAT: Enjoy right out of the fridge, or warm in a 300°F (150°C) oven for about 5 minutes.

MAKE IT WITH AN EGG: Omit the psyllium husks and replace the water and oil with one large egg; bake for only 20 minutes. You can also use your favorite plant-based egg replacer.

- Let cool in the pan for about 10 minutes, until the muffins can be carefully moved to a cooling rack. Once cool, they should easily pop out of the pan. If you used a silicone pan, run a butter knife around the inside of each well once the muffins have cooled to ensure easy removal. Garnish the muffins with red pepper flakes, if desired, before serving.

NUTRITION:
145 calories | **10.2g** fat | **7.3g** protein | **10.5g** total carbs | **3.9g** net carbs

NUTRITION (with an egg):
131 calories | **8g** fat | **8.7g** protein | **10.3g** total carbs | **4g** net carbs

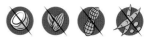

Pumpkin Spice Breakfast Bars

YIELD: 9 bars (1 per serving)

PREP TIME: 10 minutes

COOK TIME: 20 minutes

I grew up eating a lot of Nature Valley Oats 'N Honey granola bars. They were breakfasts and snacks, and even now my mom keeps a box of them at her house at all times. While these bars don't have the same flavor profile, they definitely fill that sweet-and-crunchy-snack spot that those granola bars held for me for decades.

¼ cup plus 2 tablespoons (90g) canned pumpkin puree

½ cup (80g) hulled hemp seeds

½ cup (80g) sesame seeds

¼ cup (30g) shelled pumpkin seeds (pepitas)

2 tablespoons ground flaxseed

2 teaspoons pumpkin pie spice

1 teaspoon vanilla extract

⅛ teaspoon liquid stevia

Pinch of salt

- Preheat the oven to 300°F (150°C) and line an 8-inch (40-cm) square baking pan with parchment paper. Alternatively, use a silicone pan.

- In a medium bowl, stir together all of the ingredients until completely mixed. Let the mixture sit for 5 to 10 minutes so the flax has time to set up.

- Press the seed mixture into the lined pan and spread it evenly. Using a knife, cut the uncooked seed mixture into nine equal-sized bars.

- Bake for about 20 minutes, until the bars are golden brown and firm to the touch. Let cool in the pan for about 30 minutes. Remove from the pan by slicing over your previously made cuts.

TO STORE: Keep in an airtight container in a dry place for up to 5 days.

VARIATION: Apple Bars. Substitute unsweetened applesauce for the pumpkin puree.

NUTRITION:
139 calories | **12.1g** fat | **6g** protein | **3.8g** total carbs | **1.5g** net carbs

NUTRITION (Apple Bars):
139 calories | **12.1g** fat | **5.9g** protein | **4.1g** total carbs | **1.9g** net carbs

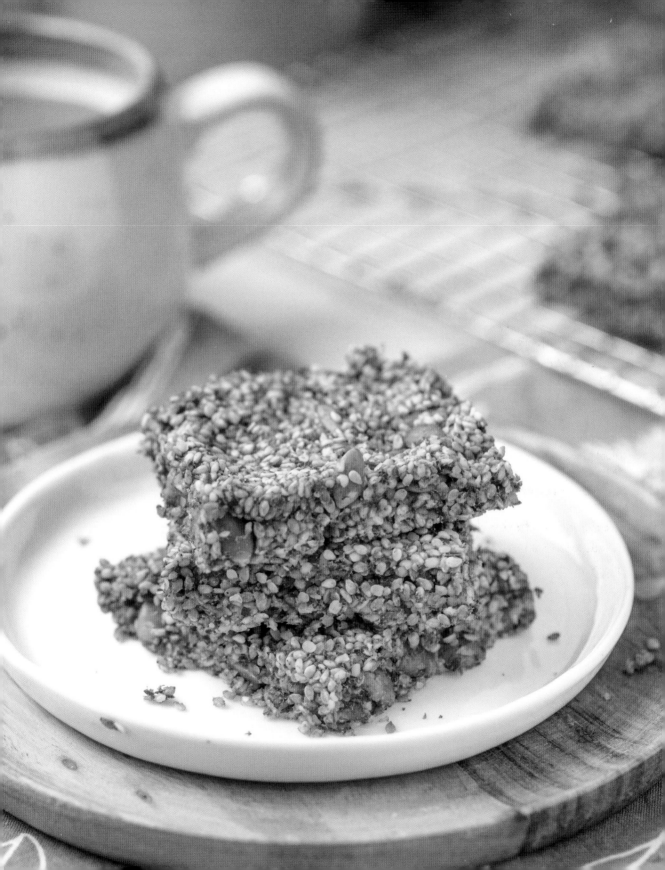

Raspberry—Beet Power Smoothie

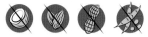

YIELD: 1 serving

PREP TIME: 5 minutes

I absolutely love beets. They're rich in vitamins, minerals, and phytonutrients, and I think they taste delicious as well. I also understand that this isn't a popular opinion—though I hope to change that! So, if the idea of beets in a smoothie is just too much, no worries at all: see the beet-free variation below.

While I usually don't add ice, it's a great way to thicken up the smoothie (and chill it even more!).

1 lightly packed cup (30g) baby spinach (see Notes)

1 cup (240ml) pea milk or other nondairy milk of choice (see Notes)

⅓ cup (30g) frozen raspberries

½ small beet (about 1 ounce/ 30g), peeled and cubed

2 tablespoons hulled hemp seeds, plus extra for garnish if desired

1 tablespoon MCT oil or coconut oil

¼ teaspoon ground cinnamon

⅛ teaspoon liquid stevia or other sweetener of choice

Ice (optional)

Put all of the ingredients in a high-powered blender and blend until completely smooth, 30 to 40 seconds. Pour into a 12-ounce (350-ml) glass to serve. Garnish with additional hemp seeds, if desired.

NOTES: I like using baby spinach in smoothies, but you can use frozen if that's what you have on hand. You can also use pretty much any green you have. I've even used lettuce that was a bit too wilted for a salad!

As for the nondairy milk, I like to use Ripple pea milk because it's high in protein, but any nondairy milk (or even water) will work. To boost the protein if using another nondairy milk or water, just add a tablespoon of your favorite sugar-free protein powder.

VARIATION: Raspberry Power Smoothie. Omit the beet and double the raspberries.

NUTRITION:
313 calories | **20.7g** fat | **17.6g** protein | **17.2g** total carbs | **5.7g** net carbs

NUTRITION (Raspberry Power Smoothie):
317 calories | **20.9g** fat | **17.5g** protein | **18.1g** total carbs | **6.1g** net carbs

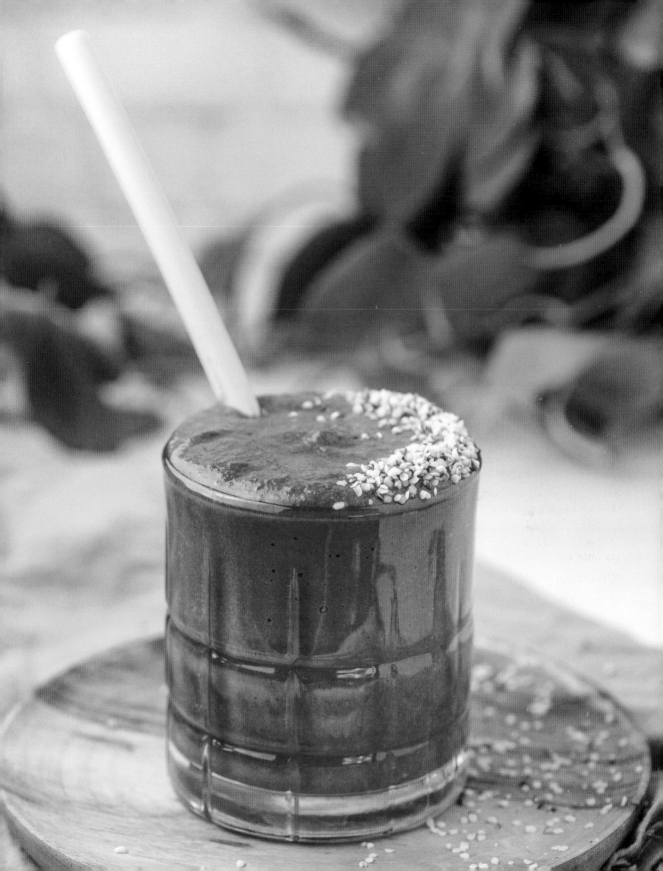

Blackberry Yogurt Smoothie Bowl

YIELD: 1 serving

PREP TIME: 5 minutes

This breakfast bowl is *dense.* It's my go-to post-workout meal these days, providing protein, fat, and carbs to help me build and preserve my (small but mighty) muscles. And yes, you read that right: because carbohydrate consumption stimulates insulin, which is anabolic, eating carbs close to a workout (either before or after) can actually help to build muscle.[50]

Because this bowl is so dense, I sometimes save half of it in the fridge for the next day.

½ **cup (120ml) coconut yogurt (see Notes)**

½ **cup (43g) frozen riced cauliflower**

⅓ **cup (50g) frozen blackberries**

¼ **cup (30g) vanilla protein powder (see Notes)**

1 **teaspoon chia seeds**

1 **teaspoon ground flaxseed**

1 **teaspoon hulled hemp seeds**

⅛ **teaspoon liquid stevia or other sweetener of choice**

Ice (optional)

SUGGESTED TOPPINGS

Fresh blackberries

Additional seeds

Cacao nibs

Chopped nuts

Unsweetened coconut flakes

Put all of the ingredients in a blender and blend until completely smooth, 2 to 3 minutes. Pour into a bowl and top as desired.

NOTES: The coconut yogurt that I use for this bowl is from Coyo or the homemade one from page 68 of my previous book, *Vegan Keto.* They're both super thick and creamy. There are plenty of other nondairy yogurts out there that you can use, though!

I used Garden of Life's raw vanilla protein powder here. For a list of other keto-friendly protein powder choices, check out page 57.

VARIATION: Raspberry Mini Smoothie Bowls. Replace the blackberries with raspberries and divide between two bowls. *Serves 2.*

NUTRITION:
494 calories | **35g** fat | **27.9g** protein | **22.7g** total carbs | **11.5g** net carbs

NUTRITION (Raspberry Mini Smoothie Bowls):
239 calories | **17.5g** fat | **13.8g** protein | **9.3g** total carbs | **4.3g** net carbs

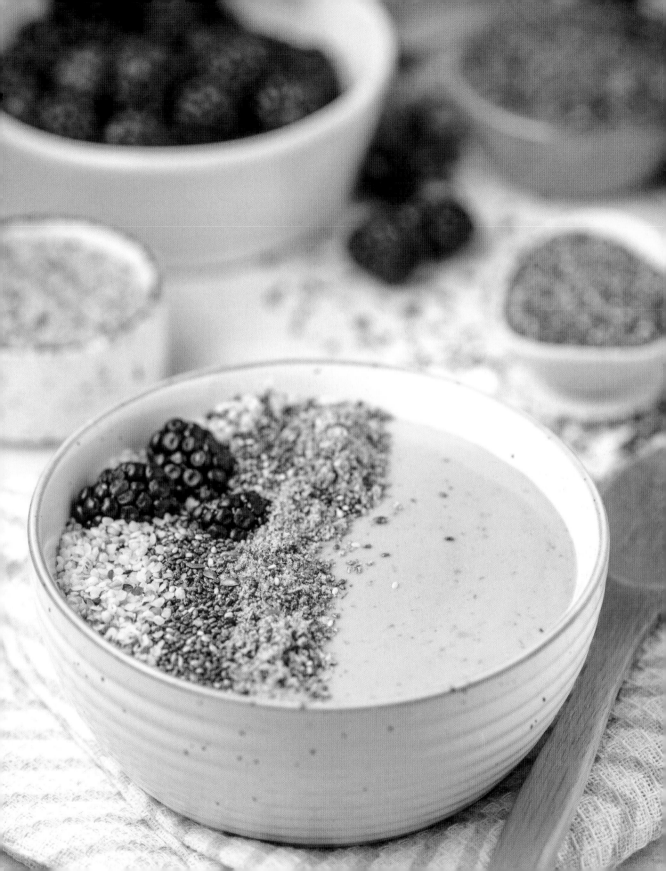

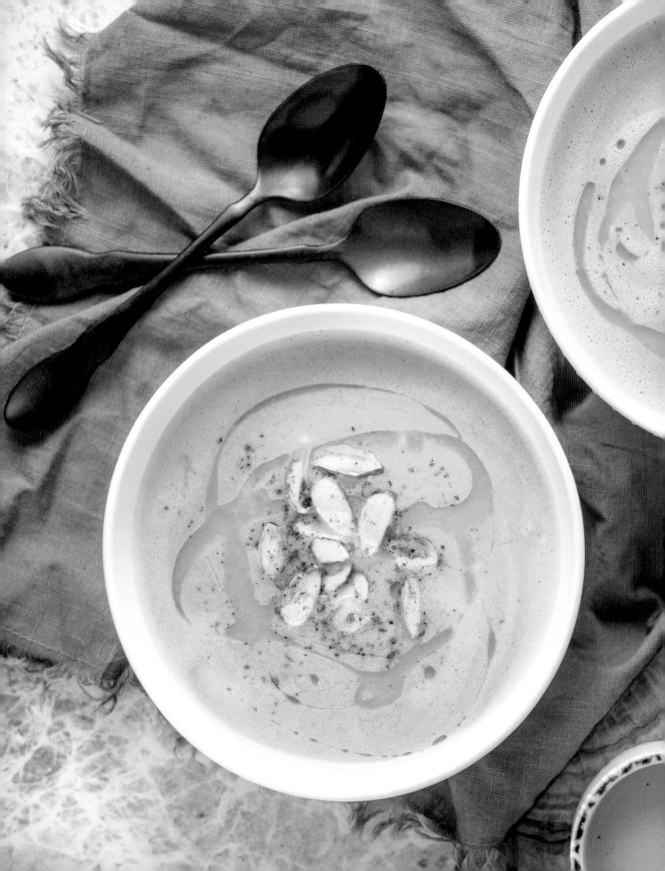

CHAPTER 2:

Soups & Salads

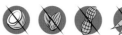

Garam Masala
Spinach Soup

YIELD: 4 servings

PREP TIME: 10 minutes

COOK TIME: 30 minutes

When I feel a cold coming on, I like to make myself a big pot of soup, specifically one loaded with fresh ginger, garlic, and some spice. This soup meets all of those qualifications, and it's delicious, too!

On days where I have more carbs to spare, this soup is yummy with a serving of chickpea pasta or RightRice (a lower-carb rice substitute made from a blend of lentils and rice).

2 tablespoons extra-virgin olive oil

2 tablespoons garam masala or curry powder blend of choice

1 tablespoon grated fresh ginger

2 teaspoons minced garlic

4 lightly packed cups (120g) fresh spinach

2 scant cups (120g) broccoli florets

3 cups (720ml) vegetable broth

1 cup (240ml) water

SUGGESTED GARNISHES

Sliced bell pepper (any color)

Chili oil

Additional seasonings

- Heat the oil in a medium soup pot or Dutch oven over medium-low heat. Add the garam masala, ginger, and garlic and cook, stirring frequently, for 1 to 2 minutes, until the ginger and garlic begin to soften.

- Add the spinach, broccoli, broth, and water and cover the pot. Simmer for about 15 minutes, until the broccoli is tender and can easily be pierced with a knife.

- Carefully pour the soup into a blender and blend until smooth, about 2 minutes. Alternatively, use an immersion blender and blend the soup directly in the pot.

- To serve, divide the soup among four bowls and garnish as desired.

TO STORE: Refrigerate in an airtight container for up to 4 days, or freeze for up to a month.

TO REHEAT: Warm in a covered saucepan over medium-low heat until the desired temperature is reached.

MAKE IT A MEAL: Add cooked black soybean noodles or Basic Baked Tofu (page 170), or top the soup with the protein topper of your choice (pages 170 to 201).

NUTRITION:
124 calories | **7.1g** fat | **2.2g** protein | **12.5g** total carbs | **3.9g** net carbs

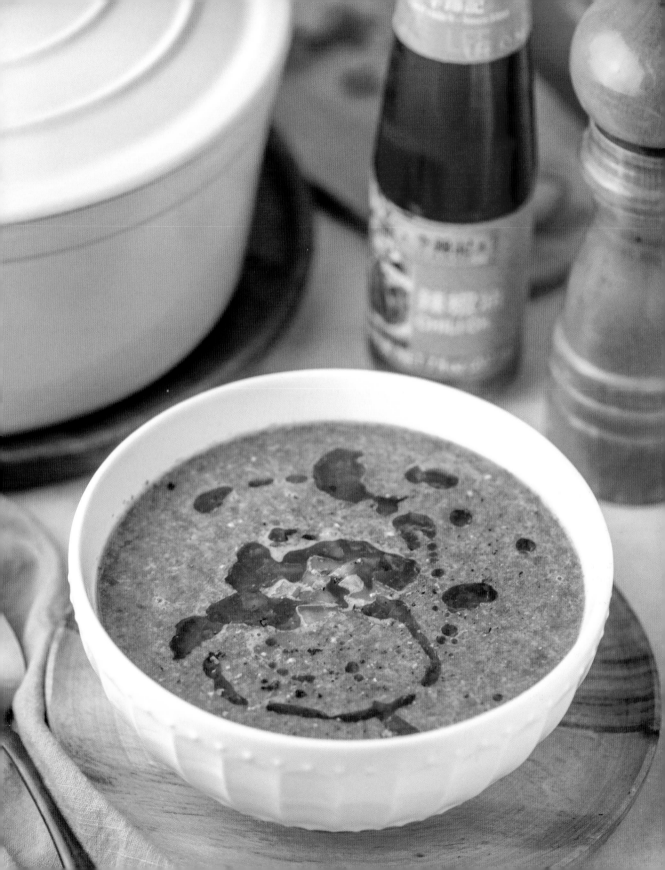

Butternut Squash Soup

YIELD: 6 servings

PREP TIME: 10 minutes

COOK TIME: 25 minutes

Squash soup just feels so cozy to me. I usually sip this soup from a mug to warm myself up on chilly days. I'll make it with whatever squash is available at the farmstand down the street, usually butternut squash or some type of pumpkin, but you can use whatever type of winter squash you like best.

If you don't have herbes de Provence on hand, you can use a poultry blend instead.

1 (13½-ounce/400-ml) can full-fat coconut milk

3 cups (720ml) vegetable broth

¾ cup (170g) cubed butternut squash

1⅔ cups (170g) roughly chopped cauliflower

2 teaspoons minced garlic

1 heaping teaspoon herbes de Provence

SUGGESTED GARNISHES

Sliced almonds (omit for nut-free)

Ground nutmeg

Drizzle of extra-virgin olive oil

- Put all of the ingredients in a large saucepan over medium heat. Cook, stirring to mix the ingredients, for about 5 minutes, until the coconut milk has melted. Cover and continue to cook until the squash and cauliflower are tender and can easily be pierced with a knife, about 20 minutes.

- Carefully pour the soup into a blender and blend until smooth, about 2 minutes. Alternatively, use an immersion blender and blend the soup directly in the pot.

- To serve, divide the soup among six bowls and garnish as desired.

TO STORE: Refrigerate in an airtight container for up to 4 days, or freeze for up to a month.

TO REHEAT: Warm in a covered saucepan over medium-low heat until the desired temperature is reached.

MAKE IT MEDIUM-CARB: Replace the cauliflower with an equal measure of butternut squash.

MAKE IT A MEAL: Top with Basic Baked Tofu (page 170) or sliced and cooked Beyond Meat brats.

NUTRITION:
134 calories | **11g** fat | **2g** protein | **7.4g** total carbs | **5.9g** net carbs

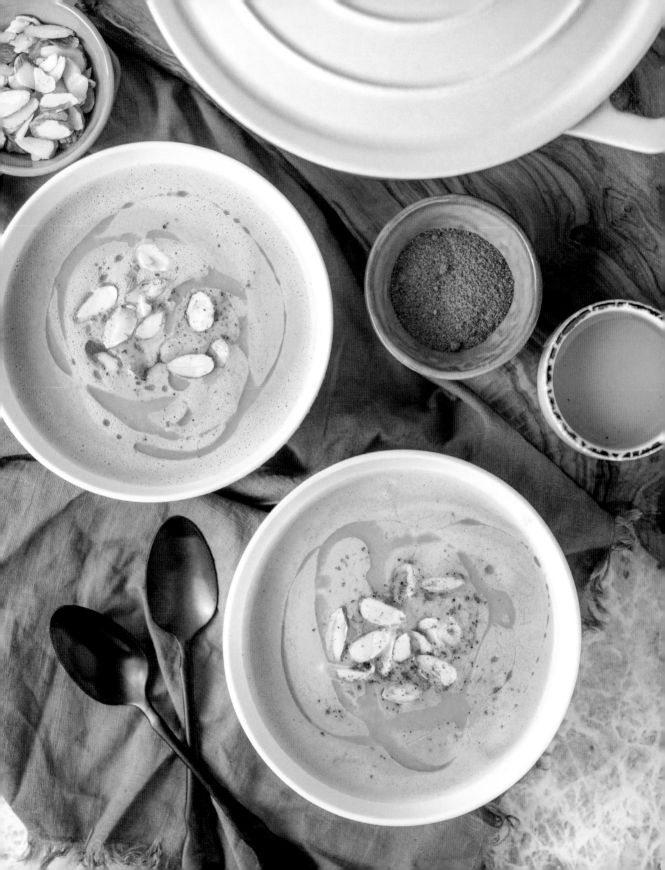

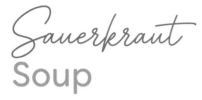

Sauerkraut Soup

YIELD: 4 servings

PREP TIME: 10 minutes

COOK TIME: 25 minutes

Sauerkraut is one of my all-time favorite foods. I put it on everything, from Lupin "Egg" Cups (page 182) to veggie burgers and even roasted vegetables. Of course, variety is the spice of life, so sometimes I like to get my sauerkraut fix in a different form. This soup has the same tanginess, with some warmth from allspice. I find it to be especially delicious on chilly winter days.

For even more depth of flavor, use mushroom broth instead of vegetable broth.

2 tablespoons extra-virgin olive oil

1 cup (100g) diced celery

¼ small onion (about 1¼ ounces/35g), diced

1 bay leaf

¼ teaspoon ground allspice

1 cup (240ml) sauerkraut

2½ cups (600ml) vegetable broth

Salt and ground black pepper

SUGGESTED GARNISHES

Chopped fresh dill

Coconut Fakon Bits (page 248)

- Heat the oil in a medium soup pot or Dutch oven over medium-low heat. Add the celery, onion, bay leaf, and allspice and cook until the vegetables are soft, about 5 minutes.

- Add the sauerkraut and broth and stir to combine. Cover and simmer for 20 minutes, until the sauerkraut is completely soft.

- Divide the soup among four bowls, season to taste with salt and pepper, and garnish as desired.

TO STORE: Refrigerate in an airtight container for up to 3 days, or freeze for up to a month.

TO REHEAT: Warm in a covered saucepan over medium-low heat until the desired temperature is reached.

MAKE IT A MEAL: Slice up a package of Beyond Meat brats and add them to the pot with the celery and onion.

NUTRITION:
82 calories | **7g** fat | **1.1g** protein | **5.1g** total carbs | **2.9g** net carbs

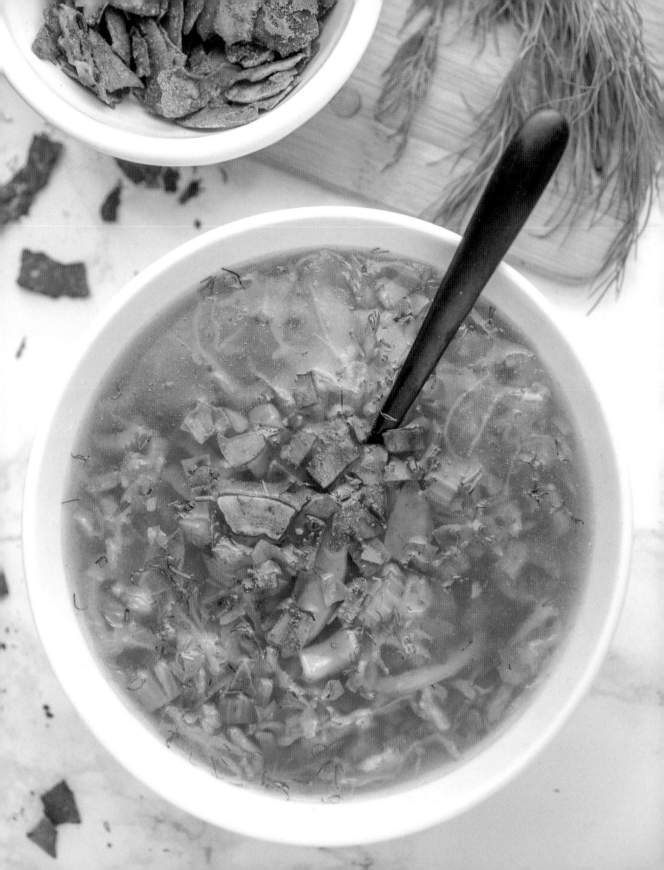

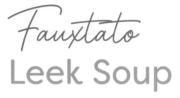

Fauxtato Leek Soup

YIELD: 4 servings

PREP TIME: 10 minutes

COOK TIME: 26 minutes

I'm so tempted to say that this soup is my favorite, but I feel like I say that about everything. Regardless, this soup is for sure in my top five. It's creamy and filling, and it's the perfect way to warm up on a chilly day.

1 medium leek

1 tablespoon coconut oil

2 cloves garlic, minced

1 (12-ounce/340-g) package riced cauliflower

2½ cups (600ml) vegetable broth

½ cup (120ml) canned full-fat coconut milk

1 teaspoon herbes de Provence

1 bay leaf

¼ teaspoon fresh cracked black pepper, plus extra for garnish

2 tablespoons sliced fresh chives, for garnish

- Prep the leek by slicing off the green leafy part and the root; quarter the remaining stalk lengthwise. Rinse the stalk well under running water (leeks are usually really sandy between the layers), then slice it crosswise.

- Heat the oil in a medium soup pot or Dutch oven over medium heat. Add the leek and cook for about 5 minutes, until softened. Stir in the garlic and cook for another minute.

- Add the riced cauliflower, broth, coconut milk, herbes de Provence, bay leaf, and pepper and stir to combine. Cover and cook for another 20 minutes, stirring occasionally, until the cauliflower has completely softened.

- Remove the bay leaf and blend the soup with an immersion blender until smooth. Alternatively, carefully pour the soup into a blender and blend until smooth.

- Divide the soup among four bowls and garnish with the chives and pepper.

TO STORE: Refrigerate in an airtight container for up to 4 days, or freeze for up to a month.

TO REHEAT: Warm in a covered saucepan over medium-low heat until the desired temperature is reached.

MAKE IT A MEAL: Top with a serving of Tempeh Bacon (page 174) and dairy-free "cheddar"—it's like a baked potato, just in soup form!

NUTRITION:
128 calories | **9.2g** fat | **2.4g** protein | **8.9g** total carbs | **7.3g** net carbs

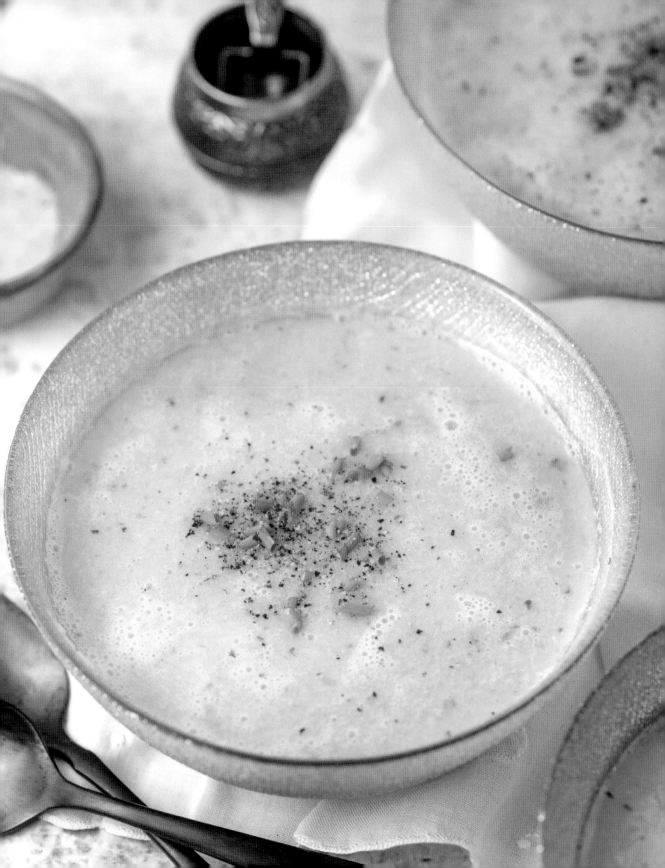

Cream of Mushroom Soup

YIELD: 3 servings

PREP TIME: 5 minutes

COOK TIME: 30 minutes

I originally came up with this soup so that I could use it in a green bean casserole that was both vegan and gluten-free. While the resulting casserole was delicious and really made my Thanksgiving meal, I also enjoy the soup on its own!

The lupin flour here functions as a thickener. If you can't find lupin flour, soy flour is another low-carb replacement. You could also use chickpea flour if you have the carbs to spare.

2 tablespoons extra-virgin olive oil

2 tablespoons minced shallot

1 teaspoon dried thyme leaves

8 ounces (225g) sliced button or cremini mushrooms

1 teaspoon salt

¼ teaspoon ground black pepper

¼ cup (30g) lupin flour

⅔ cup (160ml) canned full-fat coconut milk

2 cups (480ml) vegetable broth

Chopped fresh parsley, for garnish (optional)

- Heat the oil in a medium soup pot or Dutch oven over medium-low heat. Add the shallot and thyme and cook for 1 to 2 minutes, until the shallot has softened. Add the mushrooms, salt, and pepper and continue cooking until the mushrooms are tender, about 10 minutes more.

- Sprinkle in the lupin flour so that the mushrooms are covered. Add the coconut milk and whisk until it is absorbed by the lupin flour and a sauce starts to form. Whisk out any clumps.

- Pour in the broth and increase the heat to medium. Bring to a simmer and cook for another 15 minutes, until the mushrooms are completely soft.

- To serve, divide the soup among three bowls. Garnish with parsley, if desired.

MAKE IT MEDIUM-CARB: Replace the lupin flour with chickpea flour.

NUTRITION:
227 calories | **19.4g** fat | **7.5g** protein | **10.5g** total carbs | **5.8g** net carbs

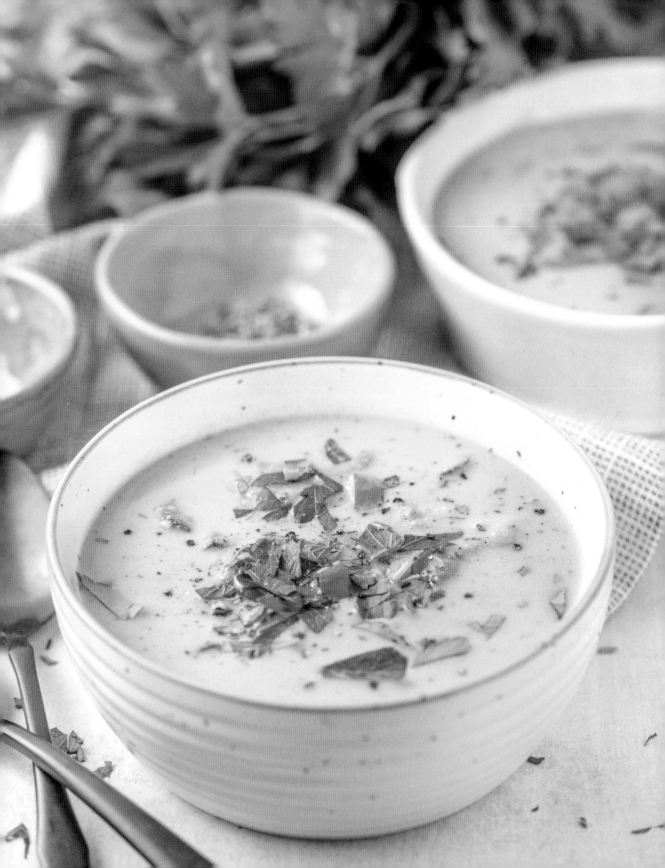

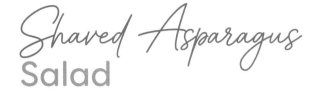
Salad

YIELD: 4 servings

PREP TIME: 10 minutes (not including time to make dressing)

One time, when I was a healthy eating specialist at a natural grocery store, I had to come up with a salad using asparagus to give away as free samples. I thought a shaved asparagus salad would be a fun idea and found a recipe that called for a pound of shaved asparagus. Well, it took me so long to prepare that I vowed never to make a shaved asparagus salad again...until I realized how tasty it was!

This is a reimagining of that salad that requires a lot less time prepping asparagus. If you've got extra time or find shaving asparagus to be calming and meditative, you can easily double the quantity without too much of a change in net carbs.

4 cups (80g) baby arugula

4 medium-thick stalks asparagus

¼ cup (60ml) Sun-Dried Tomato Dressing (page 245)

2 ounces (60g) Vegan Feta (page 180) or sheep's milk feta, crumbled

¼ cup (30g) sliced raw almonds

Ground black pepper

- Place the arugula in a large salad bowl. Trim the bottoms of the asparagus stalks and discard; cut off the tender tops and set aside for garnish. Using a vegetable peeler, shave each stalk of asparagus into the bowl.

- Drizzle the dressing over the arugula and asparagus and toss to coat. (If you do not plan to eat all of the salad right away, dress only the amount you plan to serve immediately.) Sprinkle the feta, almonds, pepper, and reserved asparagus tops over the salad and serve.

TO STORE: Refrigerate the salad and dressing separately in sealed containers for up to 3 days.

NUTRITION:
190 calories | **18.3g** fat | **3.8g** protein | **4.4g** total carbs | **2.5g** net carbs

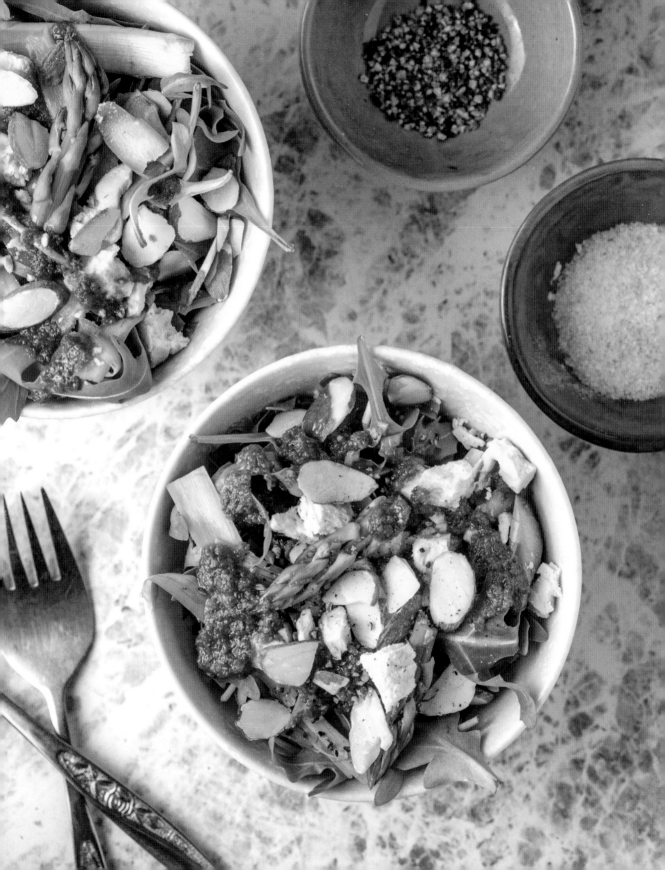

Avocado & Grapefruit
Kale Salad

YIELD: 4 servings

PREP TIME: 15 minutes

This is one of my all-time favorite salads. I started making it about a decade ago, and it's still one of my go-tos. It's so easy, but so delicious and refreshing, and it just tastes like summer. The ingredients are simple, but each one contributes a lot to the whole. Not only does the grapefruit help to tenderize the kale, but it blends nicely with the avocado, creating a somewhat creamy and tangy dressing on the leaves.

¼ **grapefruit**

6 cups (125g) chopped kale (about 1 medium bunch)

2 tablespoons minced shallot

2 medium Hass avocados (about 7½ ounces/212g), halved, pitted, and cubed

Ground black pepper

- Peel the grapefruit and remove as much of the white pith as possible. Using a paring knife, cut the thin layer of skin away on either side of each segment and remove the segments. Cut the segments into ½-inch (1.25-cm) pieces; you should have about ½ cup (115g).

- In a large salad bowl, toss together the kale, shallot, avocados, and grapefruit pieces. The grapefruit juice and avocado will mix together slightly to form a sort of dressing, with chunks of grapefruit and avocado remaining.

- Sprinkle the salad with the pepper and serve.

TO STORE: Refrigerate in an airtight container for up to 2 days.

NUTRITION:
140 calories | **11g** fat | **2.6g** protein | **11.2g** total carbs | **4.7g** net carbs

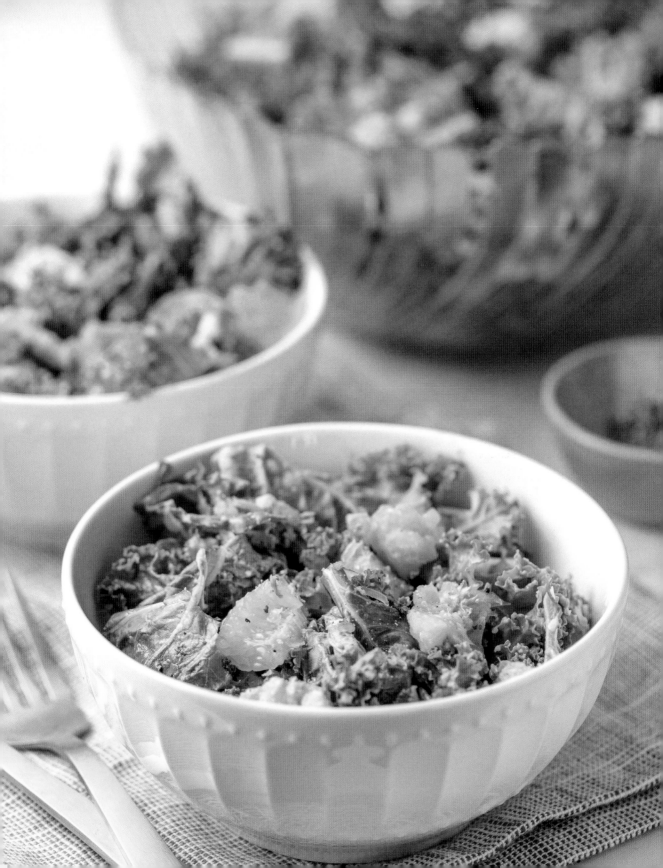

Waldorf Kale Salad

YIELD: 2 servings

PREP TIME: 8 minutes (not including time to make dressing)

This recipe, adapted from one that I used to make all the time when I worked as a healthy eating specialist, is one of my all-time favorite salads (along with the Avocado & Grapefruit Salad on page 130). Massaging the dressing into the kale makes the kale more tender and delicious and creates a nice contrast to the crunch of the jicama, celery, and walnuts.

1 recipe Walnut Dressing (page 247)

4 cups (85g) coarsely chopped kale

1 cup (100g) sliced celery

½ cup (50g) peeled and cubed jicama

¼ cup (30g) roughly chopped raw walnuts

- Place the kale in a large bowl. Pour the dressing over the kale and massage it into the leaves until they are coated. Add the celery and jicama and toss well.

- Divide the salad between two bowls and top each with half of the walnuts.

TO STORE: Refrigerate in an airtight container for up to 2 days.

MAKE IT MEDIUM-CARB: Divide ½ cup (75g) grapes between the two bowls. Or you can replace the jicama with apples or pears.

NUTRITION:
252 calories | **21g** fat | **7.1g** protein | **12.9g** total carbs | **5.1g** net carbs

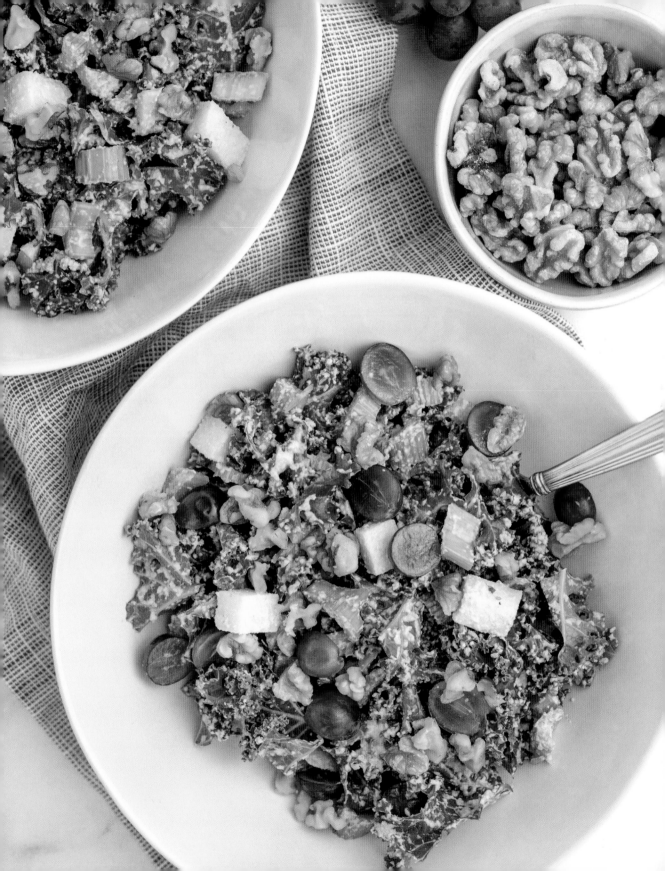

Hemp Seed Tabbouleh

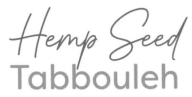

YIELD: 3 servings

PREP TIME: 15 minutes, plus 1 hour to chill

This grain-free, low-carb version of the classic Lebanese salad is a summertime favorite of mine. Every summer I grow tomatoes, cucumbers, scallions, and herbs (among other things) in a container garden on my steps, and the first thing I make when the tomatoes are ready is this salad.

If you bought your scallions from the store, you can root the white parts that aren't used in this recipe and regrow the stalks on your kitchen sill, which I think is so cool.

1 medium cucumber (about 8 ounces/225g), diced

8 ounces (225g) grape tomatoes, diced

5 scallions (green parts only), sliced

2 cups (120g) fresh parsley, roughly chopped

Leaves from 2 sprigs fresh mint

Grated zest and juice of ½ lemon

1 tablespoon extra-virgin olive oil

1 clove garlic, peeled

¼ teaspoon salt

½ cup (80g) hulled hemp seeds

- Combine the cucumber and tomatoes in a large bowl.

- Put the scallions, parsley, and mint in a food processor. Add the lemon zest and juice, oil, garlic, and salt and blend until everything is finely chopped.

- Add the herb mixture and hemp seeds to the cucumber and tomatoes and mix until completely combined. Chill for an hour before serving so the flavors have a little time to meld and the hemp seeds soak up any liquid.

TO STORE: Refrigerate in an airtight container for up to 3 days.

NUTRITION:
339 calories | **25.2g** fat | **12.7g** protein | **13g** total carbs | **7.5g** net carbs

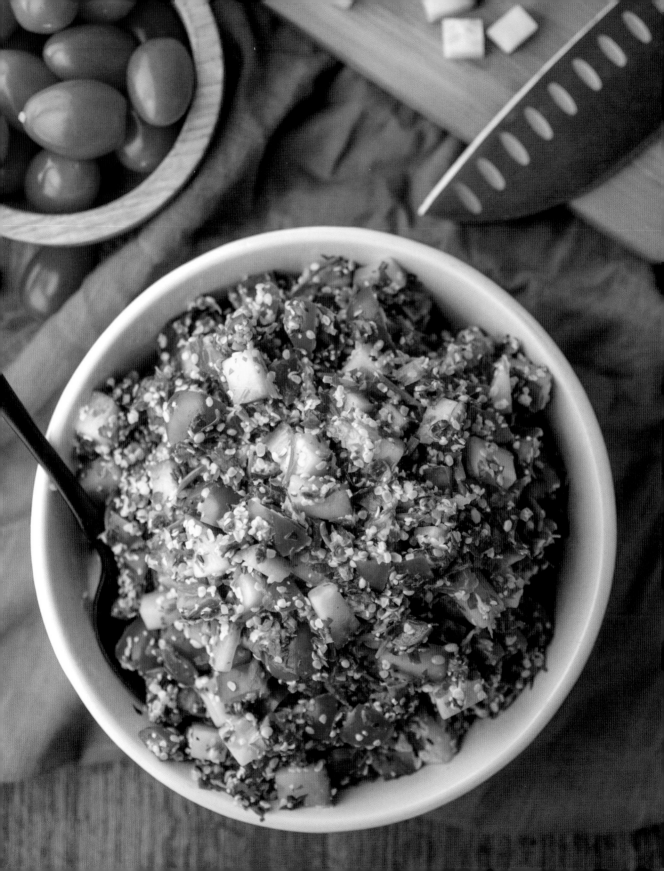

Beet Salad
with Walnut Dressing

YIELD: 4 servings

PREP TIME: 5 minutes (not including time to make dressing)

Beets are one of those vegetables that just don't get enough attention from keto dieters. Not only are they delicious, but they're also loaded with vitamins, minerals, and phytonutrients. I had a hard time deciding which dressing to use for this recipe—the walnut dressing or the balsamic—as I think they both make for delicious combinations!

5 ounces (140g) spring baby lettuce mix

1 small beet (about 2 inches/ 5cm in diameter), peeled and shredded

½ cup (60g) chopped raw walnuts

1 recipe Walnut Dressing (page 247)

2 ounces (60g) Vegan Feta (page 180), or 1 ounce (30g) sheep's milk feta or goat cheese, crumbled

Ground black pepper

Combine the lettuce, beet, walnuts, and dressing in a large salad bowl and toss until completely combined. Top with the feta and season to taste with pepper.

TO STORE: Refrigerate in an airtight container for up to 2 days.

MAKE IT MEDIUM-CARB: Add 1 cup (70g) of finely sliced purple cabbage with the lettuce, beets, walnuts, and dressing.

NUTRITION:
217 calories | **18.7g** fat | **6.9g** protein | **8.8g** total carbs | **4.9g** net carbs

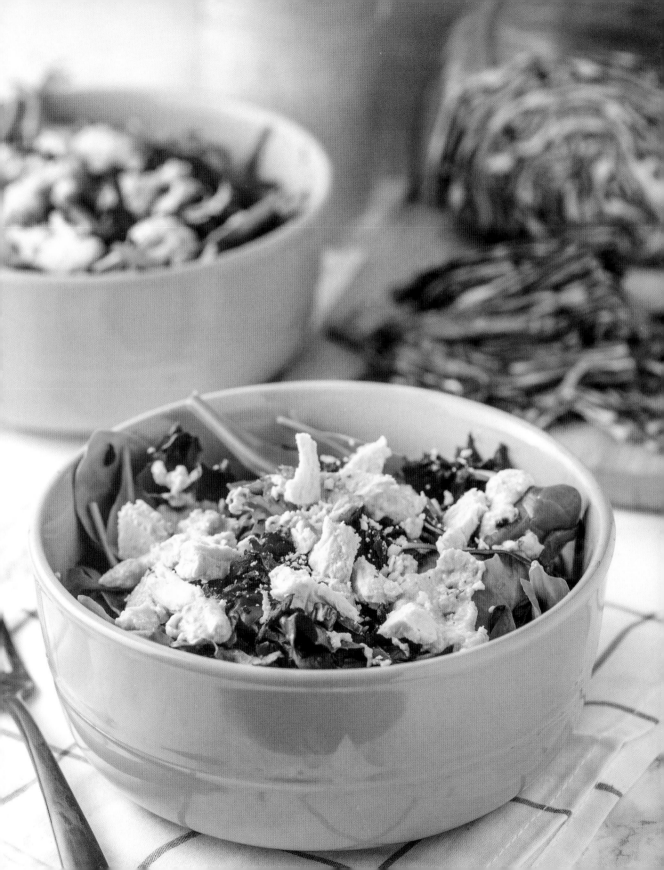

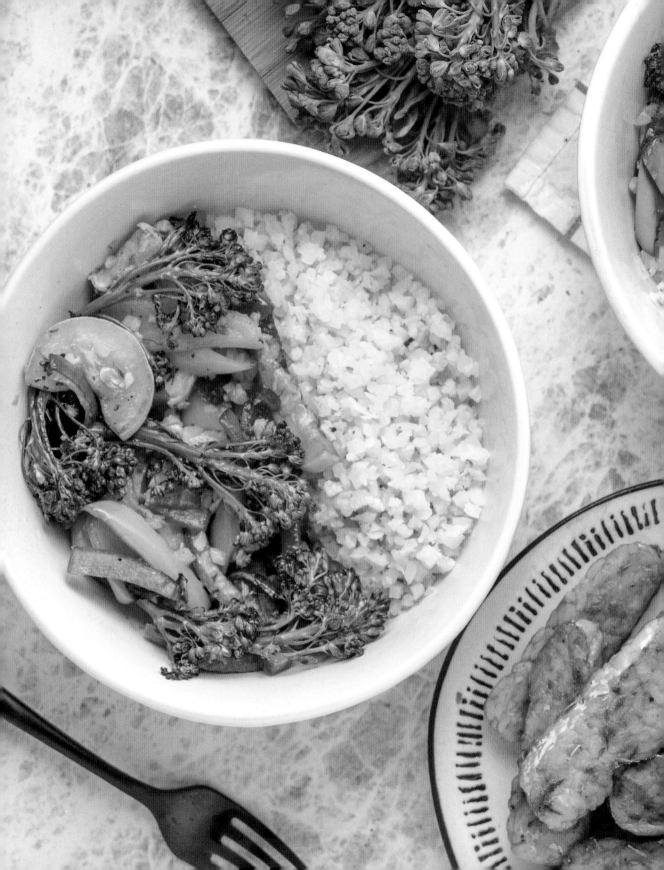

CHAPTER 3:

Entrées & Proteins

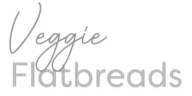

Veggie Flatbreads

YIELD: 4 servings

PREP TIME: 15 minutes, plus 15 minutes to drain squash (not including time to make toppings)

COOK TIME: 40 minutes

I used to buy premade cauliflower crusts all the time because they are so convenient. The downside is that they're kind of expensive, especially if you eat them more than once a week. So, in order to help save my wallet, I started making my own veggie crusts. I usually use zucchini because it's less work than cauliflower (no need to cook it first!), but you can definitely make these with cauliflower or broccoli rice (see Notes).

I've detailed the two topping combinations that I add most often to this crust to make veggie flatbread, but there are also plenty of days when I just scoop a bit of low-sugar marinara sauce on top and sprinkle on some nondairy cheese. I have also been known to top the flatbread with roasted garlic and chopped parsley for garlic flatbread to dip in marinara sauce. Of course, you can top these however you like!

CRUST

2 medium summer squash or zucchini (about 7 ounces/ 200g each)

¼ teaspoon salt

½ cup (32g) nutritional yeast

¼ cup (64g) tahini

¼ cup (20g) psyllium husks

SUGGESTED TOPPING COMBINATIONS

¼ cup plus 2 tablespoons (75ml) Pistachio Parsley Pesto (page 246) + 1 serving Roasted Lemon-Pepper Asparagus (page 220)

¼ cup (60ml) Sun-Dried Tomato Dressing (page 245) + 2 ounces (60g) Vegan Feta (page 180), crumbled

- Preheat the oven to 375°F (190°C) and line a rimmed baking sheet with parchment paper or a silicone baking mat.

- **To make the crust:** Grate the squash into a medium bowl and stir in the salt so that it is evenly distributed. Cover the bowl with a cloth and let sit for 15 minutes so that the salt pulls out some of the liquid. Press the liquid out using a spoon and drain it. I usually drain about ½ cup (120ml) of liquid, sometimes 1 or 2 tablespoons more.

- Stir the remaining ingredients into the squash until a uniform dough forms. Let sit for 3 to 5 minutes to thicken.

- On the lined baking sheet, press the dough into a circle, about 10 inches (25cm) in diameter and ⅛ inch (3mm) thick.

- Bake for 30 minutes, until the crust is golden brown on the bottom. Flip and bake for an additional 10 minutes, until firm and golden on both sides. Remove from the oven and carefully flip onto a cooling rack to cool completely.

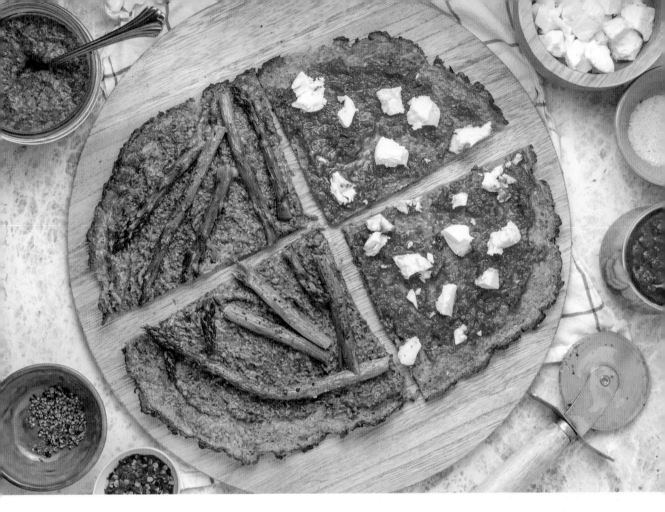

NOTES: If you can't eat (or don't like) summer squash, you can replace it with 12 ounces (340g) riced cauliflower that has been cooked until tender and drained of excess liquid. You can also make an equivalent amount of broccoli rice by processing broccoli stems in a food processor until they are the desired size (30 to 60 seconds).

If you can't decide which topping combination to use, why not split the difference for a pretty red and green pizza, as shown? Use a half quantity of the ingredients for each set of toppings.

- Turn off the oven but keep the door closed to retain the heat.

- Top the crust with the pesto and asparagus, or the dressing and feta. If you like, return the flatbread to the warm oven for 5 to 10 minutes, until the toppings are warmed through.

NUTRITION (crust only):
157 calories | **9.2g** fat | **7.4g** protein | **13.4g** total carbs | **5.4g** net carbs

NUTRITION (with Pistachio Pesto):
269 calories | **20.1g** fat | **9.2g** protein | **16.3g** total carbs | **7.1g** net carbs

NUTRITION (with Sun-Dried Tomato Dressing):
300 calories | **23.9g** fat | **8.9g** protein | **15g** total carbs | **6.6g** net carbs

Moroccan-Inspired Butternut Squash Stew

YIELD: 5 servings

PREP TIME: 10 minutes

COOK TIME: 23 minutes

When I first started making meal plans for clients, a frequent request was to convert a favorite recipe to be both vegan and keto-friendly. Usually, the client would send me scans of handwritten recipes that their mother or grandmother had given them, with notes in the margins, a light dusting of flour or spices, and a bit of sauce staining the corner. This was always my favorite part of making the plans because I could help integrate foods people already loved—which made sticking to keto a lot easier. This tagine-inspired stew is one of those recipes. It may not have all of the same ingredients as its inspiration, but the flavors are there!

The stew is delicious on its own, or you can serve it with cauliflower rice and top it with the protein of your choice (see pages 170 to 201).

3 tablespoons extra-virgin olive oil

1½ teaspoons minced garlic

1½ teaspoons grated fresh ginger

1 tablespoon ras el hanout

1 cup (200g) cubed butternut squash

1 cup (240ml) canned diced tomatoes, with liquid

1 cup (240ml) vegetable broth

1 cup (170g) jarred lupini beans (packed in brine)

¼ cup (30g) sliced raw almonds, for garnish

¼ cup (15g) chopped fresh parsley, for garnish

- Heat the oil in a large saucepan over medium-low heat. Add the garlic, ginger, and ras el hanout and cook, stirring continually, for about 3 minutes, until the garlic and ginger are fragrant, soft, and golden around the edges.

- Add the squash, tomatoes, broth, and lupini beans to the pan and place the lid slightly ajar, leaving about 1 inch (2.5cm) of space for steam to escape. Raise the heat to medium and continue to cook for 20 minutes, until the squash is tender and can easily be pierced with a knife.

- Ladle the stew into bowls, garnish with the almonds and parsley, and serve.

TO MAKE IN A PRESSURE COOKER: Put all of the ingredients except the almonds and parsley in a pressure cooker, stir to combine, and cook on high pressure for 6 minutes. Let the pressure release naturally. Ladle the stew into bowls and garnish with the almonds and parsley.

TO STORE: Refrigerate in an airtight container for up to 4 days, or freeze for up to a month.

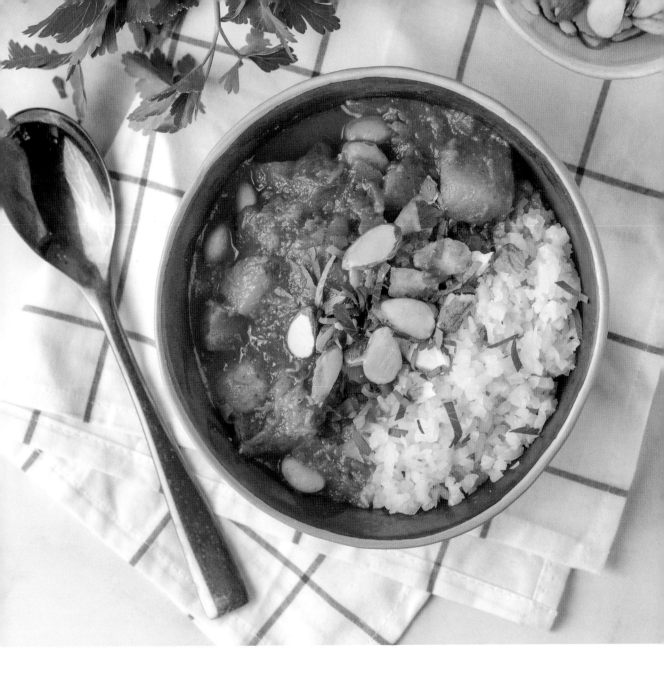

TO REHEAT: Warm in a covered saucepan over medium-low heat until the desired temperature is reached.

MAKE IT MEDIUM-CARB: Add ½ cup (65g) chopped dried apricots with the squash and replace the lupini beans with 1 cup (165g) cooked chickpeas.

NUTRITION:
190 calories | **12.2g** fat | **7.6g** protein | **13.1g** total carbs | **8.6g** net carbs

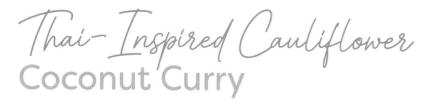

Thai-Inspired Cauliflower Coconut Curry

YIELD: 4 servings

PREP TIME: 15 minutes (not including time to make protein topper)

COOK TIME: 30 minutes

Thai is one of my favorite cuisines. Anyone who is either plant-based or gluten-free knows how hard it is to get takeout, but Thai places tend to have plenty of options that meet both of these criteria. Plus, the food always tastes amazing. Of course, once you throw keto or low-carb into the mix, eating at any restaurant can be a challenge. Often we have to come up with our own versions of our favorite dishes at home and save restaurants for special occasions. This Thai-inspired curry is my attempt at making a low-carb, plant-based dish that satisfies that craving for Thai food. Is it authentic? No, it is not. For that, you have to go to the pros.

This dish appears pretty often on my dinner table because it's easy to customize for both me and my husband (who eats both animal products and carbs). I can serve his curry over rice and mine over cauliflower rice. He usually eats the tofu but sometimes opts to cook his own protein.

2 tablespoons extra-virgin olive oil

1 small zucchini (about 4¼ ounces/120g), sliced

1 small red bell pepper (about 2½ ounces/70g), cored, seeded, and sliced

½ small onion (about 1¼ ounces/35g), sliced

¼ teaspoon salt

1 tablespoon minced garlic

1 teaspoon grated fresh ginger

2 tablespoons Thai red curry paste (see Note)

1 (13½-ounce/400-g) can full-fat coconut milk

1 pound (454g) cauliflower florets

3 scallions (green parts only), sliced, for garnish

Grated zest and juice of 1 lime, for garnish

1 recipe Super Crispy Baked Tofu (page 172) or other protein topper of choice (pages 170 to 201)

- Heat the oil in a medium frying pan over medium-low heat. Add the zucchini, bell pepper, onion, and salt. Cook, stirring occasionally, until soft, about 5 minutes.

- Add the garlic, ginger, and curry paste and cook for another minute, then pour in the coconut milk. Stir everything until completely mixed. Add the cauliflower florets, cover, and continue to cook for another 20 to 25 minutes, until the cauliflower is tender.

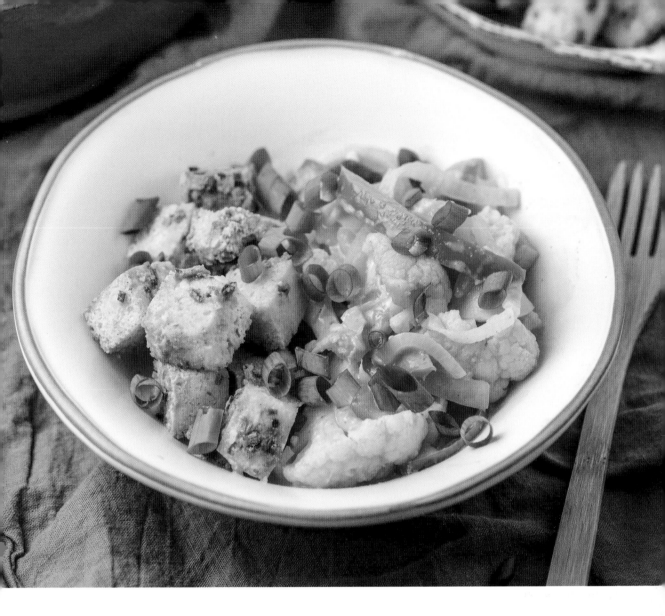

NOTE: Some brands of Thai red curry paste are vegan and others are not, so be sure to check the label if this is important to you!

TO STORE: Refrigerate in an airtight container for up to 3 days.

TO REHEAT: Warm in a preheated 300°F (150°C) oven for 5 minutes, until warmed through.

- To serve, divide among four bowls and top with scallions, lime zest and juice, and tofu or other protein.

NUTRITION (with tofu):
412 calories | **32.4g** fat | **16.4g** protein | **16.3g** total carbs | **12.2g** net carbs

NUTRITION (without protein topper):
237 calories | **20.5g** fat | **3.4g** protein | **11.1g** total carbs | **9g** net carbs

Mushroom Stroganoff

YIELD: 4 servings

PREP TIME: 5 minutes (not including time to cook squash or make protein topper)

COOK TIME: 20 minutes

Every once in a while, I'll put out a call for requests for favorite recipes to be made vegan and keto-friendly. I love the challenge of trying to capture the taste and essence of a particular dish while keeping the carbs low and using only plant-based ingredients. "Mushroom stroganoff, PLEASE!" was a request that came in over the winter, and since I'm usually eyeballs-deep in spaghetti squash in the winter (one squash plant can have such a high yield!), I decided to use that instead of noodles.

Sometimes when I make this recipe, I'll cook a package of mock ground beef with the mushrooms instead of adding a separate protein.

2 tablespoons extra-virgin olive oil

2 tablespoons minced shallot or onion

1 teaspoon dried thyme leaves

1 pound (454g) sliced button or cremini mushrooms

1 teaspoon salt

¼ teaspoon ground black pepper

½ cup (120ml) coconut cream

1½ teaspoons apple cider vinegar

2 cups (300g) cooked spaghetti squash (see Note)

1 recipe protein topper of choice (pages 170 to 201)

Chopped fresh parsley, for garnish

- Heat the oil in a large frying pan or Dutch oven over medium-low heat. Add the shallot and thyme and cook for 1 to 2 minutes, until the shallot has softened. Add the mushrooms, salt, and pepper and continue cooking until the mushrooms are tender, about 10 minutes.

- Add the coconut cream and vinegar and simmer for another 5 to 7 minutes, until the liquid has reduced by about a third. Stir in the squash until everything is well mixed.

- Top with your protein of choice, garnish with parsley, and serve.

TO STORE: Refrigerate in an airtight container for up to 3 days.

TO REHEAT: Warm in a medium frying pan over low heat until the desired temperature is reached.

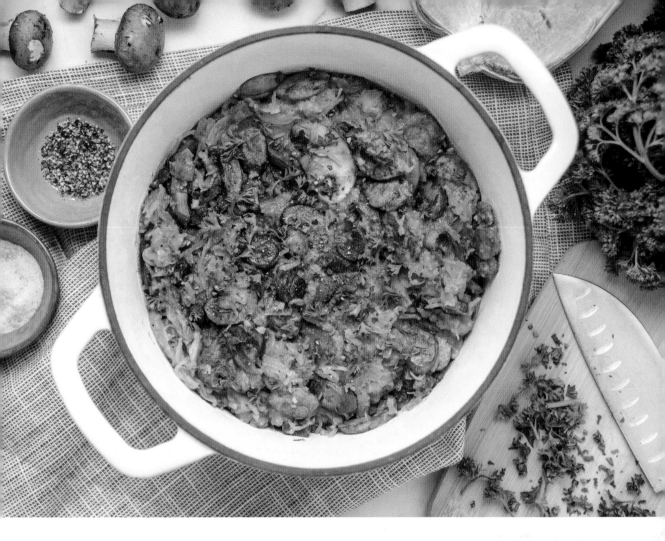

COOKING SPAGHETTI SQUASH: If you don't have cooked spaghetti squash on hand, it's easy to roast one! Preheat the oven to 375°F (190°C) and line a rimmed baking sheet with parchment paper. Carefully cut the squash in half lengthwise and scoop out the seeds with a spoon. (If you like, toss the seeds with a little oil and salt and roast them alongside the squash for a tasty snack!) Place the squash halves cut side down on the lined baking sheet and poke some holes in the tops to help release steam. Bake for about 45 minutes, until the flesh is fork-tender. Remove the squash from the oven, flip the halves over, and let cool before scraping out the "noodles" and using in the stroganoff (or another favorite pasta recipe). Refrigerate the cooked squash in an airtight container for up to 3 days.

Half of a medium spaghetti squash will yield around 2 cups of flesh.

NUTRITION (without protein topper):
160 calories | **12.4g** fat | **4g** protein | **10.2g** total carbs | **7.7g** net carbs

Greek
Stuffed Peppers

YIELD: 4 servings

PREP TIME: 10 minutes

COOK TIME: 50 minutes

A few years ago, I impulse-bought a seasoning blend with the vague name Greek Mix. It came with a few recipe suggestions, and each one turned out absolutely delicious. So I reverse-engineered the seasoning blend (see below) and started coming up with my own recipes for it. This was one of the first dishes I created, and it now makes frequent appearances on our dinner table. Sometimes in the summer, I'll make the filling and serve it in raw pepper halves instead of baking them. The peppers are nice and crunchy this way.

GREEK SEASONING
(Makes 10 tablespoons, enough for 3 batches)

¼ cup dried oregano leaves

2 tablespoons dried dill weed

2 tablespoons dehydrated onion flakes

2 tablespoons granulated garlic

1 teaspoon salt

½ teaspoon ground black pepper

2 tablespoons extra-virgin olive oil

8 ounces (225g) riced cauliflower

½ small onion, diced (about 1¼ ounces/35g)

3 tablespoons Greek Seasoning

¼ teaspoon salt

1 (8-ounce/225-g) package tempeh, or 8 ounces (225g) plant-based ground

2 ounces (56g) pitted Kalamata olives, quartered

2 large red, orange, or yellow bell peppers (about 6 ounces/ 170g each)

SUGGESTED GARNISHES

Crumbled Vegan Feta (page 180) or sheep's milk feta

Chopped fresh parsley, dill, and/or oregano

- Preheat the oven to 350°F (177°C).

- **To make the Greek seasoning:** Combine all of the ingredients in a small bowl. Measure out 3 tablespoons and store the rest in an airtight container for up to 6 months.

- Heat the oil in a medium frying pan over medium heat. Add the riced cauliflower, onion, Greek seasoning, and salt. Cook, stirring occasionally, until the veggies are soft, about 5 minutes.

- Crumble in the tempeh, stir to combine, and cook for an additional 5 minutes, until the tempeh is heated through. Remove from the heat and stir in the olives.

- Slice the peppers in half lengthwise and remove the seeds and white ribs. Divide the cauliflower mixture among the pepper halves and place on a rimmed baking sheet. Bake for 40 minutes, or until the peppers are soft. Garnish as desired and serve.

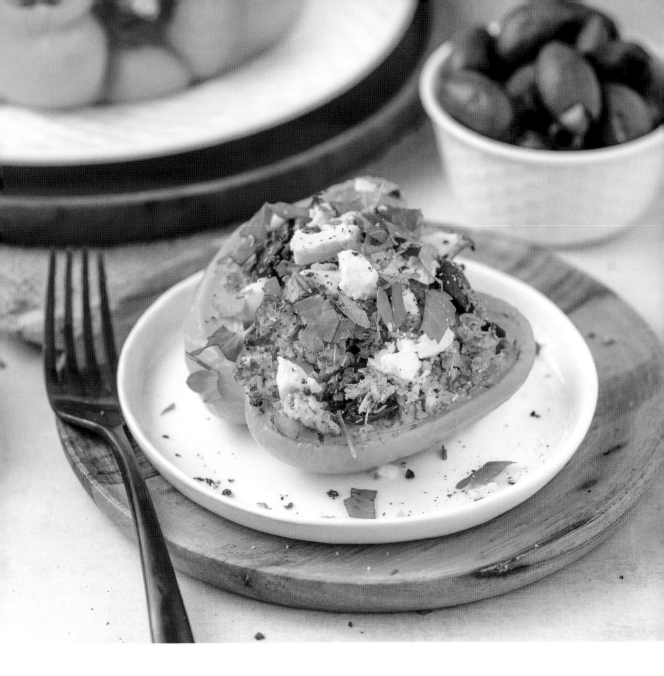

TO STORE: Refrigerate in an airtight container for up to 3 days.

TO REHEAT: Warm in a preheated 300°F (150°C) oven for 5 to 10 minutes, until warmed through.

NUTRITION (with tempeh):
243 calories | **16.6g** fat | **13.6g** protein | **14.4g** total carbs | **9g** net carbs

NUTRITION (with plant-based ground):
264 calories | **19.5g** fat | **12.1g** protein | **12.5g** total carbs | **8.2g** net carbs

Empanada-Inspired Collard Wraps

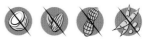

YIELD: 2 servings

PREP TIME: 20 minutes

COOK TIME: 12 minutes

Before I went raw vegan (only for a hot minute about a decade ago), I had no idea you could eat collard greens raw. I'd only had them sautéed in lots of oil with garlic and never thought to do anything else with them. That all changed when I picked up the cookbook *Raw. Vegan. Not Gross.* by Laura Miller, which uses collard leaves as wraps. It sounds silly, but it blew my young mind, and I have not stopped using greens as wraps since. (Chard also makes a great wrap!)

The word *empanada* roughly translates as "wrapped in bread," so you are not wrong if you think it's odd that there is no bread in sight here. But trust me on this: collard greens are super nutrient-dense and delicious!

If you're feeling fancy, toss in some chopped olives; and for a higher-carb option, toss in some raisins.

2 tablespoons extra-virgin olive oil

¾ cup (64g) riced cauliflower

½ small onion, diced (about 1¼ ounces/35g)

½ small red bell pepper (about 1¼ ounces/35g), cored, seeded, and sliced

¼ teaspoon salt

2 teaspoons minced garlic

2 teaspoons dried thyme leaves

1½ teaspoons chili powder

1 teaspoon smoked paprika

⅛ teaspoon ground black pepper

8 ounces (225g) plant-based ground (see Note)

4 large collard leaves

Chimichurri (page 242), for dipping (optional)

- Heat the oil in a medium frying pan over medium-low heat. Add the riced cauliflower, onion, bell pepper, and salt and cook, stirring occasionally, until soft, about 5 minutes. Add the garlic, thyme, chili powder, paprika, and black pepper and cook for another minute before adding the plant-based ground. Stir well, making sure the mock meat is fully combined with the vegetables. Continue cooking for another 5 minutes, until the mock meat is heated through, then remove from the heat.

- Prep the collards by washing them and removing some of the large vein that runs down the middle of each leaf, leaving the top third in the leaf.

- Spread a collard leaf flat on a clean work surface and spoon one-quarter of the filling mixture in a line across the top of the

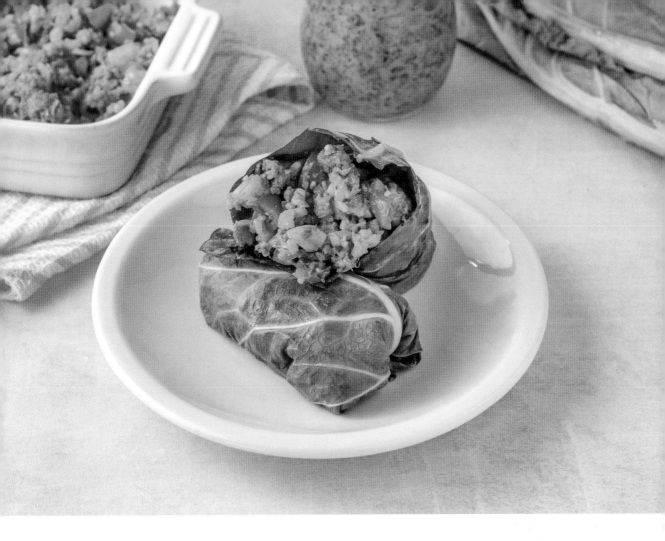

NOTE: Any brand of ground beef–style mock meat will work, or you can use ground meat if you eat animal products. You can also use an equal measure of crumbled tempeh or 1 cup (120g) walnuts soaked in near-boiling water for a half hour and then chopped.

VARIATION: EMPANADA-INSPIRED SALAD: Instead of wrapping the filling in collard leaves, serve it over 4 lightly packed cups (120g) mixed baby greens (or whatever salad greens you like best) and top with 2 tablespoons chimichurri as a dressing.

leaf, making sure to leave at least 1 inch (1.25cm) of space for wrapping. Starting at the sides, fold the edges of the leaf around the filling, then wrap the rest of the leaf to make sort of a collard burrito. Place the wrap seam side down on a plate. Repeat with the remaining leaves and filling, making a total of four wraps.

- Slice the wraps in half and serve with chimichurri for dipping, if desired.

NUTRITION:
343 calories | **25.7g** fat | **22.6g** protein | **11.8g** total carbs | **6.7g** net carbs

NUTRITION (Empanada-Inspired Salad):
348 calories | **25.7g** fat | **22.9g** protein | **12.7g** total carbs | **7.1g** net carbs

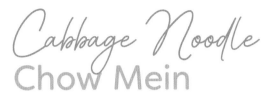
Cabbage Noodle Chow Mein

YIELD: 4 servings

PREP TIME: 10 minutes (not including time to make protein topper)

COOK TIME: 25 minutes

If this dish looks oddly familiar, that's because it's based on a very specific one from a very specific panda-themed takeout restaurant here in the States. When I make it at home, I'll make myself a batch of Basic Baked Tofu and sometimes fry up an egg or two for my husband.

I find that adding just a bit of Chinese five-spice lends the sweetness and richness of oyster sauce without the actual sugar...or the oysters. I also like using white pepper here, but if you have only black pepper, you can use it instead.

3 tablespoons extra-virgin olive oil

2 (8-ounce/225-g) packages shirataki noodles (see Note), thoroughly rinsed and drained

½ small onion (about 1¼ ounces/35g), thinly sliced

½ cup (50g) thinly sliced celery

3 tablespoons low-sodium tamari

¼ teaspoon Chinese five-spice powder

Pinch of ground white pepper

4 cups (280g) shredded green cabbage

1 recipe Basic Baked Tofu (page 170) or other protein topper of choice (pages 170 to 201)

Chopped fresh parsley, for garnish (optional)

- Heat the oil in a large frying pan over medium heat. Add the noodles and cook until completely dry, about 5 minutes. They will likely make a hissing noise: this process helps with the taste and texture.

- Add the onion, celery, tamari, five-spice powder, and pepper and cook, stirring constantly, for 5 minutes, until the celery and onion have browned slightly. Add the cabbage and continue cooking until it is soft, another 15 minutes.

- Top with the tofu or other protein, garnish with parsley, if desired, and serve.

NOTE: If you cannot tolerate shirataki (konjac) noodles, you can use spiral-sliced zucchini or daikon radish instead. Or you can omit them and double the shredded cabbage.

TO STORE: Refrigerate in an airtight container for up to 4 days.

TO REHEAT: Warm in a small frying pan over low heat until the desired temperature is reached.

NUTRITION (with tofu):
290 calories | 22g fat | 13.7g protein | 12.8g total carbs | 7.5g net carbs

NUTRITION (without protein topper):
130 calories | 10.2g fat | 2.5g protein | 9g total carbs | 5g net carbs

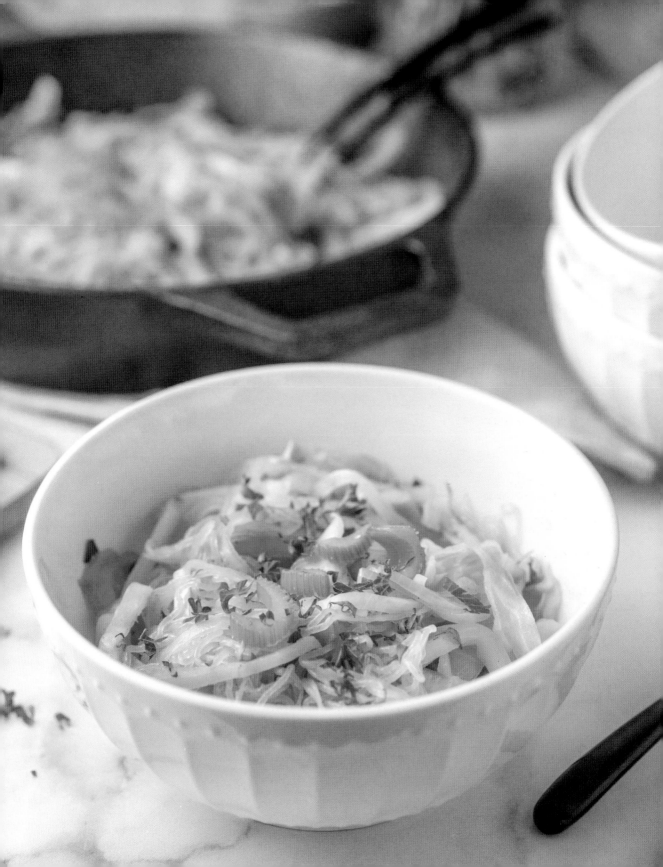

Lemony Noodles with Peas & Edamame

YIELD: 2 servings

PREP TIME: 5 minutes (not including time to make optional protein topper)

COOK TIME: 12 minutes

My favorite kinds of meals are those that are nutrient-dense and full of veggies, but also easy and not too time-consuming to make. This noodle bowl meets all of those requirements! If I'm having this dish for lunch, I usually don't bother adding a protein, but when I make it for dinner, I find that Basic Baked Tofu (page 170) is a great protein boost. Toss the tofu in the oven and then start making the noodles, and both should be done around the same time.

To make this dish soy-free, simply omit the edamame and top the noodles with Mushroom "Meatballs" (page 178) or another soy-free protein topper.

2 tablespoons extra-virgin olive oil

2 tablespoons lemon juice

1 teaspoon minced garlic

½ cup (80g) frozen shelled edamame

¼ cup (40g) frozen peas

¼ cup (16g) nutritional yeast, or ¼ cup (25g) grated Parmesan cheese, plus extra for garnish

2 cups (200g) zucchini noodles (about 1 medium zucchini)

Salt and ground black pepper

1 recipe protein topper of choice (pages 170 to 201) (optional)

Grated lemon zest, for garnish (optional)

- Heat the oil, lemon juice, and garlic in a medium frying pan over medium-low heat. Once the garlic begins to soften, add the edamame and cook for about 5 minutes, until the beans are tender.

- Add the peas, nutritional yeast, and zucchini noodles and stir to coat the noodles evenly. Reduce the heat to low and continue to cook for another 2 to 3 minutes, until the noodles are just tender and the peas are warmed through.

- Season with salt and pepper to taste, top with a protein topper, if desired, garnish with lemon zest, and serve.

TO STORE: Refrigerate in an airtight container for up to 2 days.

TO REHEAT: Warm in a small frying pan over low heat until the desired temperature is reached.

NUTRITION (without protein topper):
233 calories | **16.3g** fat | **10.5g** protein | **13.7g** total carbs | **8.2g** net carbs

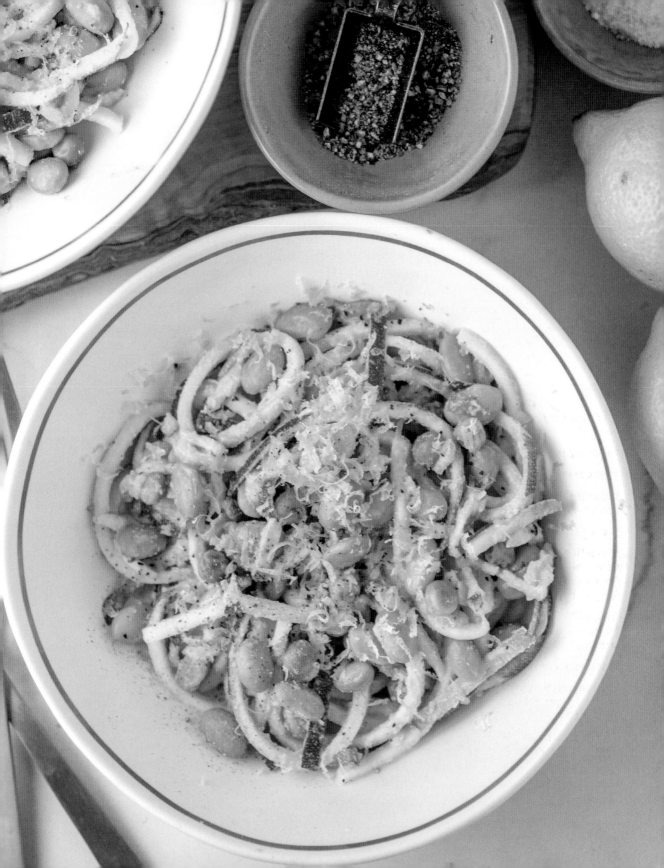

Pan-Fried Gnocchi with Garlicky Kale

YIELD: 2 servings

PREP TIME: 15 minutes, plus 30 minutes to chill dough

COOK TIME: 15 minutes

Who doesn't love dumplings, especially when they're pan-fried? Gnocchi are traditionally made with potato, egg, and wheat flour—all ingredients that can be used as a binder. These plant-based gnocchi include exactly none of those ingredients. Are they still gnocchi? Whether or not they qualify as gnocchi, they are delicious and high in protein. If you have some wiggle room carb-wise, I highly recommend topping the gnocchi and kale with marinara sauce.

GNOCCHI

4 ounces (112g) silken tofu

½ cup (60g) lupin flour

¼ cup (28g) coconut flour

2 tablespoons tahini

¼ teaspoon baking powder

¼ teaspoon salt

2 tablespoons extra-virgin olive oil, divided

4 cups (85g) baby kale

2 teaspoons minced garlic

Salt and ground black pepper

SUGGESTED GARNISHES

Nutritional yeast

Red pepper flakes

TO STORE: Refrigerate in an airtight container for up to 3 days.

TO REHEAT: Warm in a small frying pan over low heat until the desired temperature is reached.

- **To make the gnocchi:** Mash all of the gnocchi ingredients together, then knead until a firm and slightly tacky dough forms, about 3 minutes. There should be no remaining flour visible. If there is, work in some water, 1 tablespoon at a time, until the dough is uniform. Wrap in plastic wrap or parchment paper and chill for at least 30 minutes.

- Using a pastry bag or a zip-top bag with a corner cut off, pipe 1-inch (2.5-cm) dumplings and place them in a bowl or on a plate. Alternatively, scoop up ½-tablespoon portions and roll into oblong shapes.

- Using a pastry brush, spread 1 tablespoon of the oil in a large frying pan and heat over medium-low heat. Add the gnocchi, cover, and cook for 8 minutes, until they firm up and are just golden on the bottom. Continue cooking, shaking the pan so that the gnocchi move around, for another 2 minutes, until the gnocchi are firm and just starting to turn golden on the other side. Transfer the gnocchi to a medium bowl.

- Pour the remaining 1 tablespoon of oil into the pan. Add the kale, garlic, and a sprinkle of salt and pepper and cook, stirring occasionally, for 2 minutes, until the kale just starts to wilt. Return the gnocchi to the pan, stir everything together, and cook, uncovered, for a final minute. Remove from the heat, garnish as desired, and serve.

NUTRITION:
329 calories | 21.3g fat | 22.1g protein | 24.5g total carbs | 6.1g net carbs

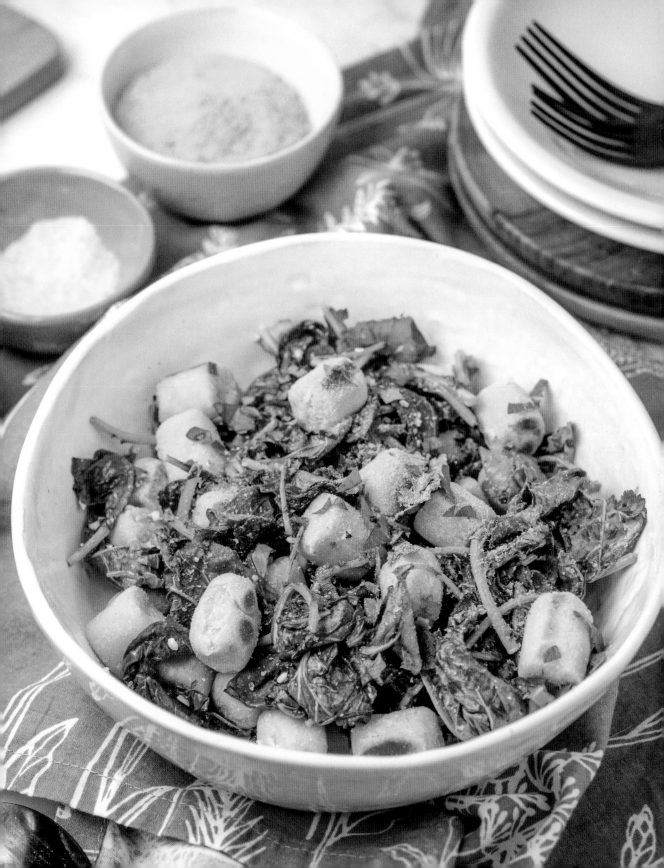

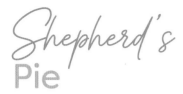

Shepherd's Pie

YIELD: 4 servings
PREP TIME: 20 minutes
COOK TIME: 50 minutes

When I ask my husband what he wants for dinner, at least half the time he will say shepherd's pie. When we first started dating, I made it with real potatoes, but over time, I've sneaked more and more cauliflower into the mix, and now I just make it with cauliflower mash and he doesn't even blink.

The brand of plant-based ground that I usually use is Beyond Meat. It's very low in carbs and doesn't contain any soy or gluten. If you're not a fan of Beyond Meat (or have trouble finding it), other brands should work just fine.

1 pound (454g) cauliflower florets

2 tablespoons dairy-free buttery spread or extra-virgin olive oil

¼ teaspoon plus ⅛ teaspoon salt, divided

1 tablespoon sliced fresh chives

1 tablespoon extra-virgin olive oil

½ cup (50g) diced celery

½ small onion (about 1¼ ounces/35g), diced

¼ cup (30g) diced carrots

¼ teaspoon ground black pepper

1 (1-pound/454-g) package plant-based ground

TO STORE: Refrigerate in an airtight container for up to 3 days.

TO REHEAT: Warm in a preheated 300°F (150°C) oven for 5 minutes, until warmed through.

- Preheat the oven to 350°F (177°C).

- Cook the cauliflower in a pot of boiling water until fork-tender, about 10 minutes. Drain and transfer to a blender or food processor. Add the buttery spread and ⅛ teaspoon of the salt and blend until smooth. Remove the blade, stir in the chives, and set aside.

- Heat the oil in a medium frying pan over medium heat. Add the celery, onion, carrots, pepper, and remaining ¼ teaspoon of salt and cook, stirring occasionally, until the vegetables begin to soften, about 5 minutes.

- Add the plant-based ground to the pan, breaking up any large clumps. Stir well, incorporating the mock meat into the vegetable mixture so everything is completely combined. Continue cooking for another 5 minutes, until the mock meat is heated through, then remove from the heat.

- Spread the mock meat and vegetable mixture evenly in the bottom of a 2-quart (2-liter) casserole dish, then spread the cauliflower mixture on top, smoothing out any peaks.

- Bake for 25 to 30 minutes, until the cauliflower mash starts to turn lightly golden. Remove from the oven and let cool for about 10 minutes before serving.

NUTRITION:
316 calories | **22.1g** fat | **22.9g** protein | **12.3g** total carbs | **7.2g** net carbs

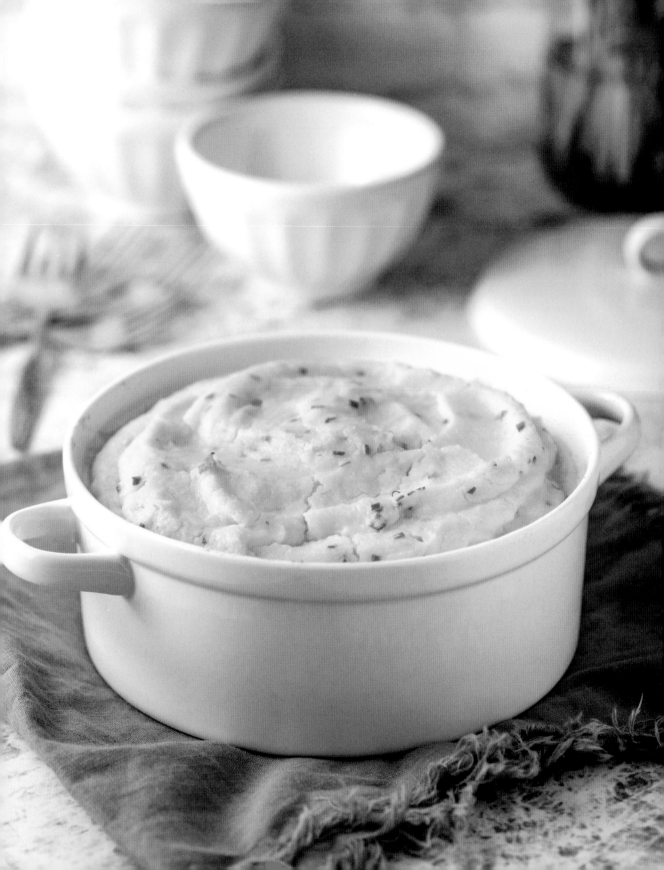

Korma-Inspired Cauliflower Bake

YIELD: 4 servings

PREP TIME: 10 minutes

COOK TIME: 35 minutes

Don't be alarmed by the number of ingredients here! I don't usually make recipes with more than ten ingredients (or even more than seven or eight) because my brain gets overwhelmed by seeing a list that it perceives as too long, and I sort of freeze up. The same thing happens when there are loads of steps. I know I'm not alone in this! However, I promise that this recipe is not complicated. Most of the ingredients just get blended together for the sauce.

This dish is a simplified ketogenic version of the vegetable korma from my favorite Indian takeout restaurant, with a protein boost from hemp seeds. While it's not the same as the original, it certainly hits the spot until I can enjoy some takeout on a higher-carb day!

SAUCE

1 cup (160g) hulled hemp seeds

⅔ cup (160ml) canned full-fat coconut milk

⅓ cup (80ml) water

1 tablespoon lemon juice

1 tablespoon minced garlic

1 tablespoon grated fresh ginger

1 tablespoon tomato paste

2 tablespoons garam masala (see Note)

1 teaspoon turmeric powder (optional)

1 teaspoon smoked paprika

¾ teaspoon salt

¼ teaspoon ground black pepper

1 pound (454g) cauliflower florets

1 small carrot (about 1¾ ounces/50g), sliced

SUGGESTED GARNISHES

¼ cup (30g) sliced raw almonds

Chopped fresh cilantro or parsley

- Preheat the oven to 375°F (190°C) and grease a 13 by 9-inch (33 by 23-cm) or 2-quart (2-liter) baking dish.

- **To make the sauce:** Blend all of the sauce ingredients in a blender or food processor until completely smooth and creamy, 2 to 3 minutes.

- In a large bowl, mix the sauce with the cauliflower florets and carrots. Transfer the mixture to the greased baking dish and bake for 35 minutes, until the cauliflower is tender and can easily be pierced with a knife.

- Garnish with the almonds and cilantro, if desired, and serve.

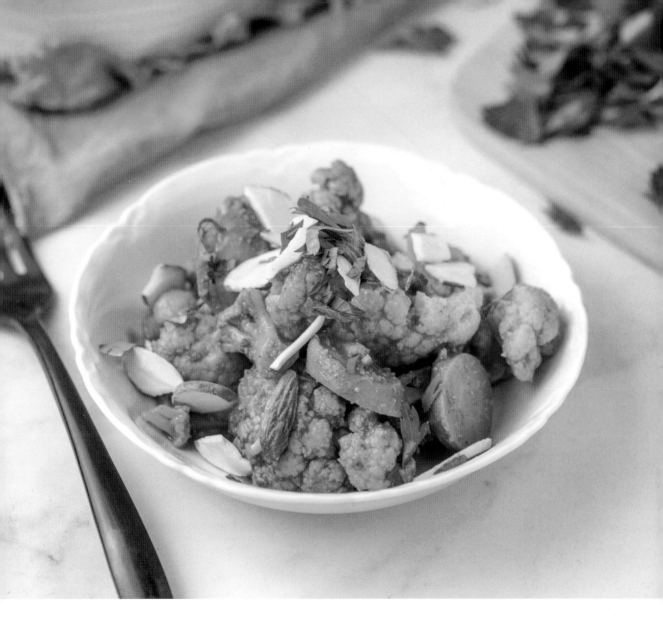

NOTE: Garam masala—a name for a warming spice blend that typically contains fennel, cloves, cinnamon, pepper, cardamom, and ground chiles (among many other ingredients, depending on the region)—isn't usually too spicy, but if you really don't like heat, you may want to start by blending just 1 tablespoon into the sauce and tasting it before adding more.

TO STORE: Refrigerate in an airtight container for up to 3 days, or freeze for up to a month.

TO REHEAT: Heat in a preheated 300°F (150°C) oven for 10 to 15 minutes (or 25 to 30 minutes if frozen), until warmed through.

MAKE IT MEDIUM-CARB: Double the carrots and add 1 cup (150g) peas.

NUTRITION:
364 calories | **25.9g** fat | **18.3g** protein | **20.6g** total carbs | **12.5g** net carbs

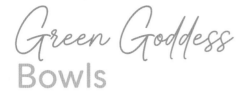

Green Goddess
Bowls

YIELD: 2 servings

PREP TIME: 15 minutes (not including time to make dressing)

You know how each color has its own feeling? Well, to me, all greens feel like life and health and energy. Light green feels especially exuberant and filled with youthful zest. This veggie bowl is basically the food embodiment of green—not only in color, but also in the physical feelings. This is one of those meals that gets me so jazzed up after eating, like when you have a particularly good green smoothie and you feel like each one of your cells is more awake and alive. I hope this meal also makes you feel bright and ready to take on the world!

1 medium cucumber (about 7 ounces/200g), spiral-sliced into noodles

1 cup (30g) chopped baby spinach

1 cup (155g) shelled cooked edamame

1 cup (100g) sliced celery

1 medium Hass avocado (about 7½ ounces/212g), halved, pitted, and sliced

½ cup (120ml) Green Goddess Dressing (page 241)

¼ cup (40g) hulled hemp seeds

2 scallions (green parts only), sliced

Red pepper flakes (optional)

Divide the cucumber noodles, spinach, edamame, celery, and avocado cubes between two bowls and top each bowl with half of the dressing, hemp seeds, and scallions. Sprinkle with red pepper flakes, if desired.

MAKE IT SOY-FREE: Replace the edamame in each bowl with a serving of Mushroom "Meatballs" (page 178) or another protein topper of your choice (pages 170 to 201).

TO STORE: Refrigerate without dressing in an airtight container for up to 3 days.

NUTRITION:
439 calories | **34g** fat | **19.1g** protein | **23.2g** total carbs | **9.9g** net carbs

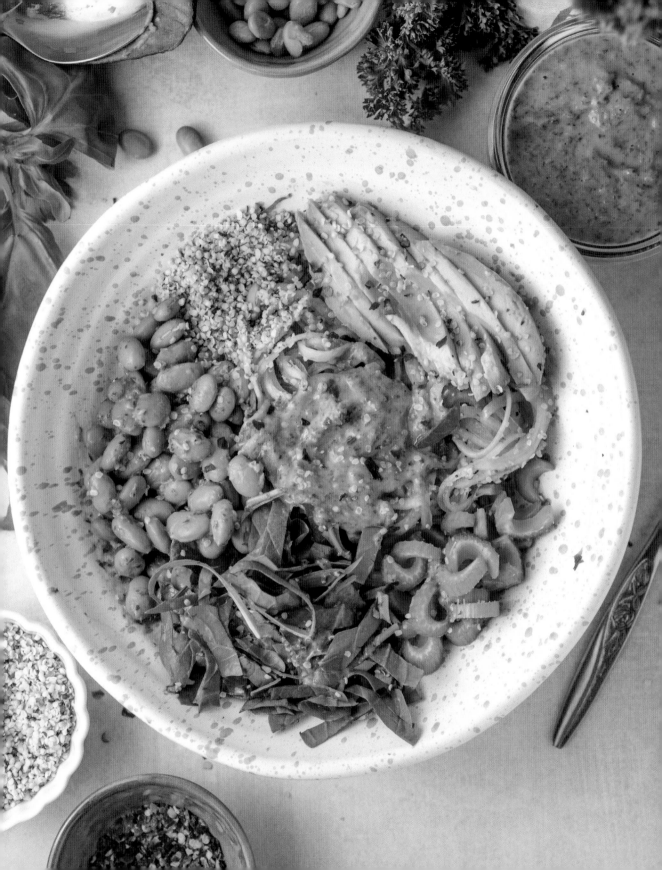

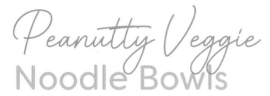
Peanutty Veggie Noodle Bowls

YIELD: 2 servings

PREP TIME: 5 minutes (not including time to make sauce or optional protein topper)

If you want a meal that is filling, delicious, nutrient-dense, and ready in less than 10 minutes, you are in luck! While I say the prep time is 5 minutes, that is a generous estimate. It really is so fast to make. This is one of my favorite dinners in the summer when I don't even want to look at the stove, never mind actually turn it on. Sometimes I'll add some protein (I really like tossing some cooked mock chicken on this), but a lot of the time I just enjoy it on its own.

If you aren't a fan of zucchini noodles, this bowl is also delicious with daikon radish noodles or carrot noodles, though keep in mind that carrots are higher in carbs.

8 ounces (225g) zucchini noodles

¼ cup plus 2 tablespoons (90ml) Pantry Peanut Sauce (page 243)

½ cup (60g) raw peanuts, coarsely chopped

2 scallions (green parts only), sliced

¼ teaspoon red pepper flakes

1 recipe protein topper of choice (pages 170 to 201), optional

- Put the noodles in a large bowl. Pour the dressing and half of the peanuts over the noodles and toss well.

- Divide the noodles between two serving bowls and top each with half of the remaining peanuts, scallions, and red pepper flakes. Top with a protein topper, if desired.

TO STORE: Refrigerate in an airtight container for up to 2 days. The sauce will soften the zucchini noodles in the fridge, so if you prefer your noodles crunchy, store them separately.

NUTRITION:
323 calories | **25.8g** fat | **14.8g** protein | **14.5g** total carbs | **8.6g** net carbs

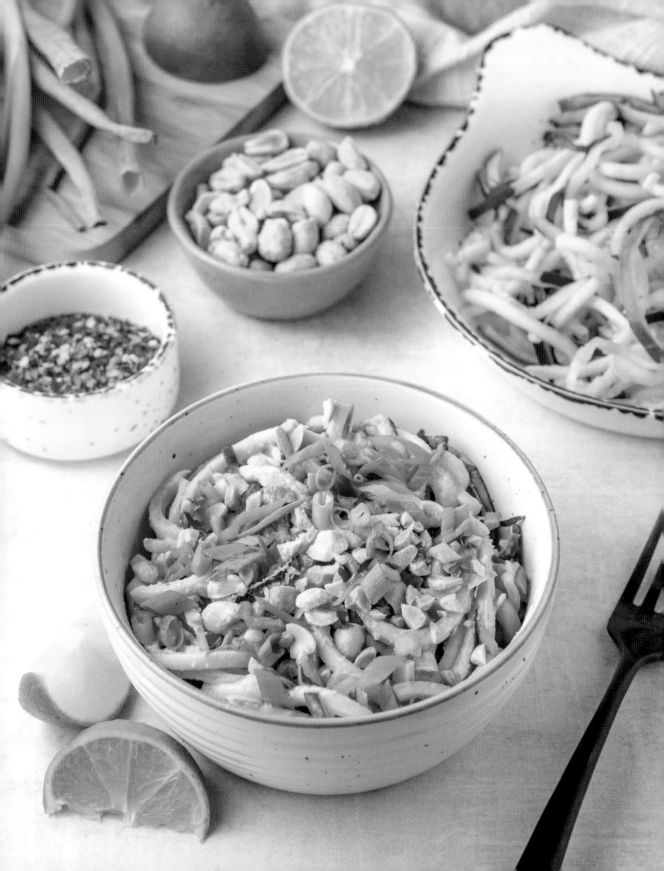

Balsamic Roasted
Veggie Bowls

YIELD: 2 servings

PREP TIME: 15 minutes (not including time to make vinaigrette or protein topper)

COOK TIME: 25 minutes

Did you know you can roast riced cauliflower? It's a total game changer, not only because roasting adds another layer of flavor and texture to a sometimes boring dish, but also because you can stick it in the oven and then not think about it for 25 minutes. Win-win.

I like making veggie bowls as a way to use up those little bits of vegetable that are hanging around in the fridge, and this one is a great way to use up a lot of scraps that accumulate throughout the week, especially since peppers, onions, and summer squash make so many appearances on my dinner table.

If you don't want to make your own balsamic vinaigrette, I understand. Store-bought is totally fine!

1½ cups (107g) riced cauliflower

1½ teaspoons extra-virgin olive oil

3½ ounces (100g) broccoli rabe florets or broccoli florets

½ small red onion (about 1¼ ounces/35g), sliced

½ small yellow, orange, or red bell pepper (about 1 ounce/25g), cored, seeded, and sliced

½ cup (75g) sliced summer squash or zucchini

2 tablespoons Balsamic Vinaigrette (page 244)

¼ teaspoon dried thyme leaves

Pinch of salt

Pinch of ground black pepper

2 servings Balsamic-Marinated Skillet Tempeh (page 176) or other protein topper of choice (pages 170 to 201)

- Preheat the oven to 425°F (220°C) and line a rimmed baking sheet with parchment paper or a silicone baking mat.

- In a large bowl, toss the riced cauliflower with the oil, then spread on one half of the lined baking sheet.

- In the same bowl, toss the broccoli rabe, onion, bell pepper, and squash with the vinaigrette, thyme, salt, and black pepper. Spread the vegetables on the other half of the baking sheet.

- Roast for 20 to 25 minutes, stirring each portion of vegetables after about 10 minutes, until the vegetables are tender and starting to crisp around the edges.

- To serve, divide the cauliflower rice and vegetables between two bowls and top with the tempeh or other protein of choice.

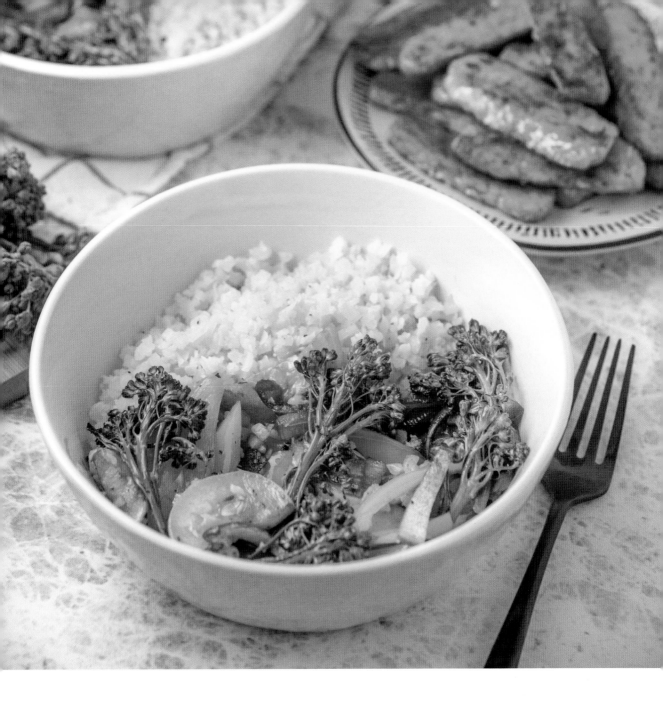

TO STORE: Refrigerate in an airtight container for up to 4 days.

TO REHEAT: Enjoy leftovers cold, or warm in a small frying pan over low heat until the desired temperature is reached.

<u>NUTRITION:</u>
417 calories | **32.5g** fat | **14.6g** protein | **21.9g** total carbs | **2.6g** sugar alcohols | **8.8g** net carbs

<u>NUTRITION (without protein topper):</u>
176 calories | **14.2g** fat | **4.4g** protein | **10.5g** total carbs | **6.3g** net carbs

Broccoli Noodle Bowls with Peanut Sauce

YIELD: 2 servings

PREP TIME: 15 minutes (not including time to make sauce)

COOK TIME: 15 minutes

Do you ever make a meal so delicious that you want to eat it every day? This is that meal for me. It's such a simple set of ingredients, but to me, it's a magical combination. I make this dish at least once a week, and some weeks I have it almost every day. I usually rotate between the garnishes listed, sometimes opting for a little more chili oil and other times just scallions.

If you don't care for black soybean noodles, you can use pretty much any noodle in their place—zucchini, shirataki, and kelp noodles all work well. My favorite substitution, though, is daikon radish noodles (made by spiral-slicing daikon radish). I leave them raw for some crunch!

2 ounces (56g) black soybean noodles (see Note)

2 tablespoons toasted sesame oil

8 ounces (225g) bite-sized broccoli florets

¼ cup (25g) chopped yellow, orange, or red bell pepper

Pinch of salt

6 tablespoons (90ml) Pantry Peanut Sauce (page 243)

1 tablespoon sesame seeds

SUGGESTED GARNISHES

Red pepper flakes

Sliced scallions (green parts only)

Lime juice

Chili oil

- Cook the noodles according to the manufacturer's directions. Divide the cooked noodles between two serving bowls.

- Heat the sesame oil in a large frying pan over medium heat. Add the broccoli and bell pepper, sprinkle with the salt, and stir-fry until the broccoli is tender, about 10 minutes.

- Divide the broccoli and bell pepper between the two bowls. Top each bowl with 3 tablespoons of the dressing and half of the sesame seeds. Garnish as desired and serve.

NOTE: Black soybean pasta is one of my absolute favorite wheat noodle substitutes. Not only is it low in carbs, but it packs a ton of protein into a small serving. The noodles also have a nice texture that's pretty close to actual pasta. They're widely available, to the point that I can even buy them at T.J. Maxx!

TO STORE: Refrigerate the bowl ingredients and the dressing in separate airtight containers for up to 3 days. Enjoy leftovers cold.

NUTRITION:
405 calories | **28.8g** fat | **22.6g** protein | **22.5g** total carbs | **10.7g** net carbs

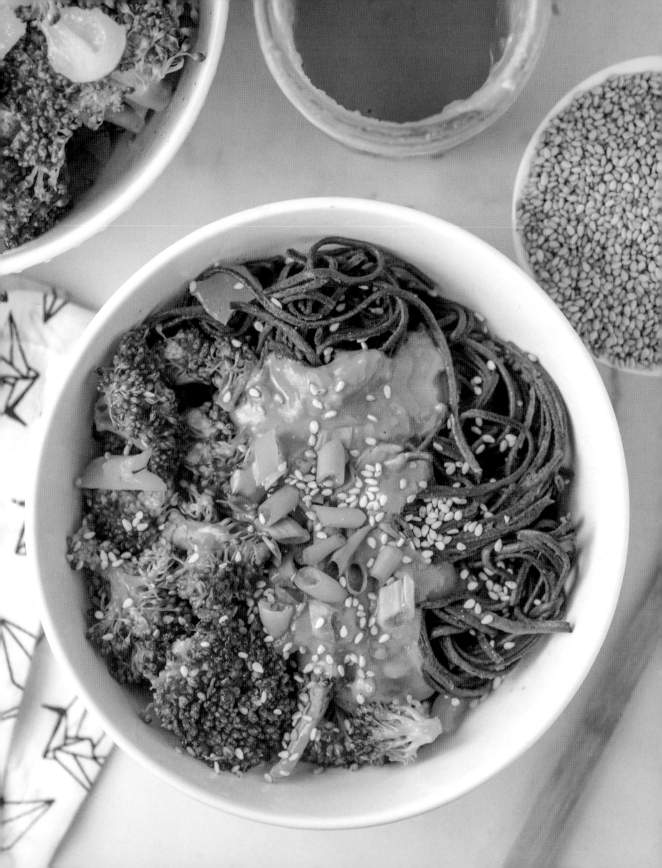

Basic Baked Tofu

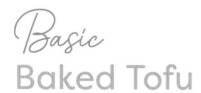

YIELD: 4 servings

PREP TIME: 5 minutes

COOK TIME: 15 minutes

If you have only 20 minutes to get dinner on the table, this is the tofu for you. The beautiful thing about tofu is that it's more or less a blank canvas. I have yet to find a flavor profile that doesn't work! I have listed two of my favorite variations below, but you can really customize this recipe for any seasoning combination.

1 (14-ounce/397-g) block extra-firm tofu

2 tablespoons extra-virgin olive oil

¼ teaspoon salt

⅛ teaspoon ground black pepper

- Preheat the oven to 425°F (220°C) and line a rimmed baking sheet with parchment paper.

- Drain the block of tofu and press out any excess liquid. Cut the tofu into ¾-inch (2-cm) cubes.

- In a large bowl, whisk together the oil, salt, and pepper. Toss the tofu cubes in the oil mixture until they are completely coated.

- Spread the tofu cubes on the lined baking sheet and bake for 15 minutes, or until crispy around the edges.

TO STORE: Refrigerate in an airtight container for up to 4 days.

TO REHEAT: Warm in a preheated 300°F (150°C) oven for about 5 minutes, until warmed through.

VARIATIONS:

Lemon Pepper Baked Tofu. Whisk the oil with the grated zest of 1 lemon, ¼ teaspoon salt, and ¼ teaspoon ground black pepper and toss with the cubed tofu.

Mediterranean Baked Tofu. Whisk the oil with 1 teaspoon smoked paprika, ½ teaspoon ground cumin, ½ teaspoon granulated onion, ½ teaspoon granulated garlic, ¼ teaspoon salt, and ¼ teaspoon ground black pepper and toss with the cubed tofu.

NUTRITION:
160 calories | **11.7g** fat | **11.3g** protein | **3.8g** total carbs | **1.3g** net carbs

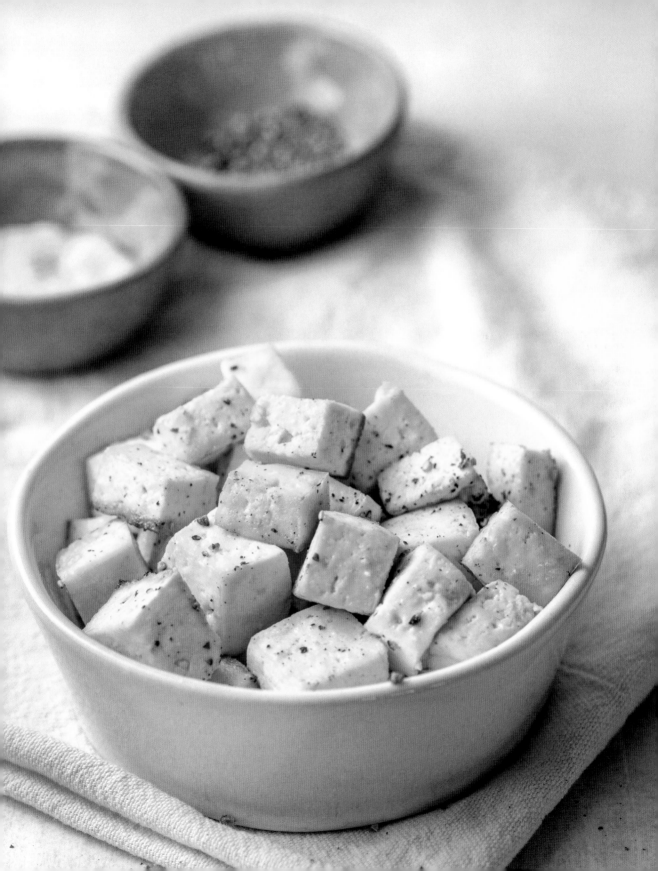

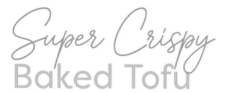
Super Crispy
Baked Tofu

YIELD: 4 servings

PREP TIME: 5 minutes

COOK TIME: 25 minutes

Back in the olden days, when I was inhaling carbs like they were oxygen, I used to make my crispy tofu using cornstarch. While it was delicious and certainly very crispy, it was also very starchy, and thus carby. So I sought a replacement. I tried bean flours, nut flours, coconut flour, and probably others that I no longer remember. Some of them turned out okay, but none achieved the crispiness I was looking for. Until one day, purely by accident, I discovered that the key to deliciously crispy tofu had been under my nose the whole time—nutritional yeast.

Pro tip: I once asked a chef friend how he got his tofu to be so chewy, and he told me the easiest and most game-changing trick ever: freeze the block of tofu in the packaging overnight and then thaw it before using it in a recipe. You'll be able to press out the liquid easily once it thaws. If you don't have time to do this, that's fine! This tofu will still be delicious. But freezing really takes the texture to the next level.

1 (14-ounce/397-g) block extra-firm tofu

2 tablespoons extra-virgin olive oil

¼ cup (16g) nutritional yeast

¼ teaspoon salt

⅛ teaspoon ground black pepper

- Preheat the oven to 425°F (177°C) and line a rimmed baking sheet with parchment paper.

- Drain the block of tofu, press out any excess liquid, and pat dry with a clean cloth. Cut the tofu into ¾-inch (2-cm) cubes.

- In a large bowl, whisk together the oil, nutritional yeast, salt, and pepper. Toss the tofu cubes in the oil mixture until they are completely coated.

- Spread the tofu cubes on the lined baking sheet and bake for 25 minutes, or until super crispy, crunchy, and golden.

TO STORE: Refrigerate in an airtight container for up to 4 days.

TO REHEAT: Warm in a preheated 300°F (150°C) oven for about 5 minutes, until warmed through.

VARIATIONS:

Garlic-Chive Super Crispy Baked Tofu. Whisk 1 tablespoon dried chives and 2 teaspoons garlic powder into the oil mixture.

Chili-Lime Super Crispy Baked Tofu. Whisk 1 tablespoon chili paste or Sriracha sauce and the grated zest and juice of 1 lime into the oil mixture.

NUTRITION:
175 calories | **11.9g** fat | **13g** protein | **5.3g** total carbs | **3.3g** net carbs

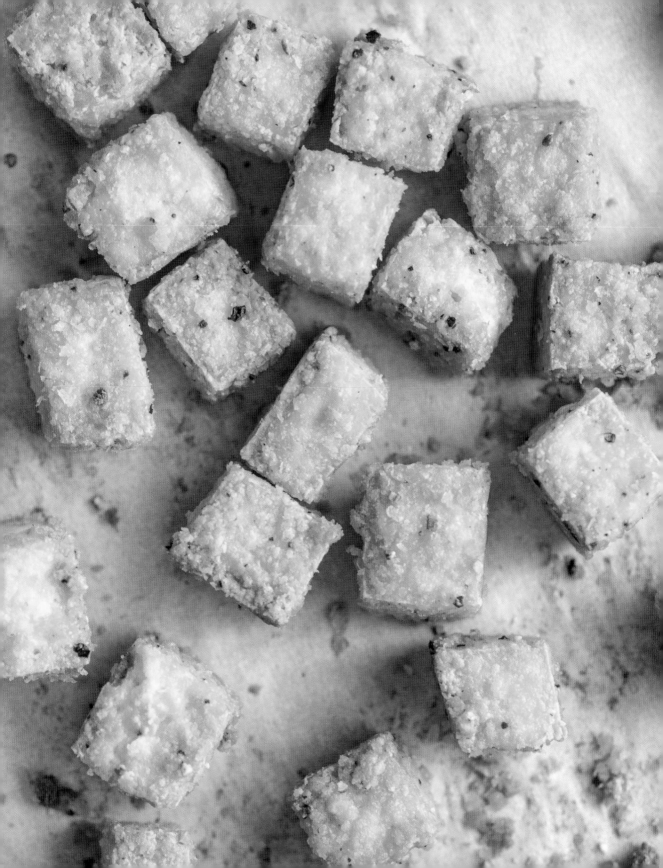

Tempeh Bacon

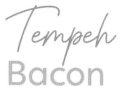

YIELD: 4 servings

PREP TIME: 5 minutes, plus 30 minutes to marinate

COOK TIME: 20 minutes

Tempeh is a great source of protein that takes on other flavors really well. While you could use tofu for this recipe, I prefer tempeh's denser texture.

An important thing to note about tempeh is that some varieties contain a lot of grains, and thus more carbohydrates. Definitely check the nutrition information on the package! The types I buy have only 1 to 2 grams of net carbs per serving, but I've seen some that are as high as 6 grams.

If you don't eat soy, many brands now offer soy-free tempeh. My favorite, made from hemp seeds, is appropriately called *hempeh.*

2 tablespoons low-sodium tamari

2 tablespoons sugar-free maple syrup

1 tablespoon extra-virgin olive oil

½ teaspoon smoked paprika

1 (8-ounce/225-g) package tempeh

TO MAKE IN AN AIR FRYER: Lay the marinated tempeh slices in a single layer on the air fryer tray and cook for 15 minutes at 375°F (190°C), until crispy.

TO STORE: Refrigerate in an airtight container for up to 4 days.

TO REHEAT: Warm in a preheated 300°F (150°C) oven for about 5 minutes, until warmed through.

- In a medium food storage container with a lid, whisk together the tamari, maple syrup, oil, and paprika.

- Cut the block of tempeh into ¼-inch (6-mm) slices and place them in the tamari mixture. Secure the lid of the container, hold it down tightly, and gently shake to cover the tempeh in the mixture. Chill in the refrigerator for 30 minutes, gently shaking the container every 10 minutes to redistribute the marinade.

- Preheat the oven to 375°F (190°C) and line a rimmed baking sheet with parchment paper.

- Arrange the tempeh slices on the lined baking sheet. Brush or pour the remaining marinade over the tempeh.

- Bake for 20 minutes, or until crispy around the edges. Enjoy warm.

NUTRITION:
163 calories | **8.8g** fat | **13.1g** protein | **8.8g** total carbs | **1.3g** sugar alcohols | **2.1g** net carbs

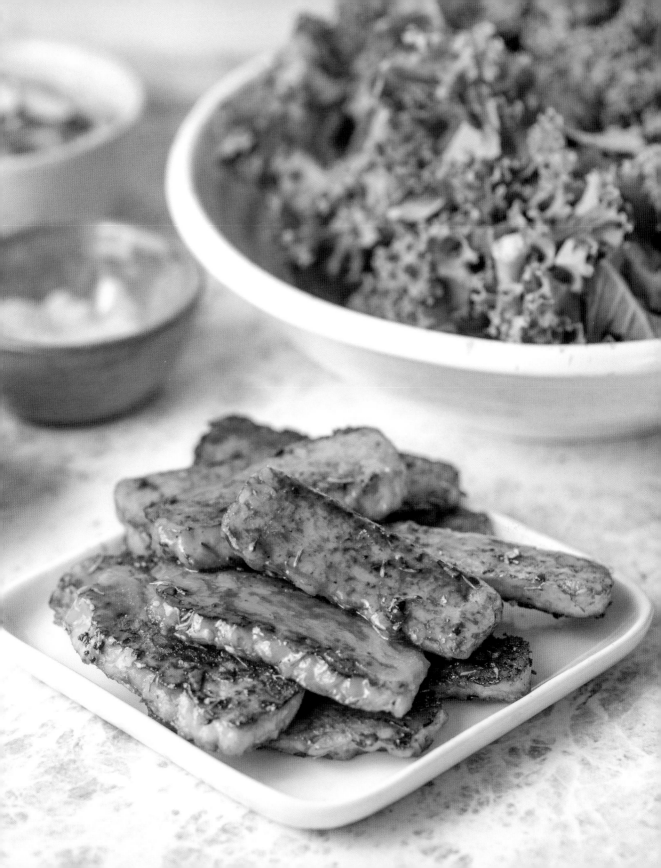

Balsamic-Marinated Skillet Tempeh

YIELD: 4 servings

PREP TIME: 5 minutes, plus 30 minutes to marinate (not including time to make vinaigrette)

COOK TIME: 5 minutes

When I first started eating tempeh, I had no idea what to do with it. It was unlike anything I had ever cooked, and it just seemed really weird (though it's hard to say how much of that can be attributed to the fact that I was a teenager, so everything seemed weird). In time, tempeh became a regular in my rotation of fridge staples, in part because of easy recipes like this one.

¼ cup (60ml) Balsamic Vinaigrette (page 244)

2 tablespoons sugar-free maple syrup

1 (8-ounce/225-g) package tempeh, cut into ¼-inch (6-mm) slices

1 tablespoon extra-virgin olive oil

- In a medium bowl, whisk together the vinaigrette and maple syrup. Add the tempeh, making sure the pieces are submerged. Marinate in the refrigerator for at least 30 minutes, gently shaking the container every 10 minutes to redistribute the marinade.

- Heat the oil in a medium frying pan over medium heat. Using tongs, place the tempeh pieces in the oil, reserving the marinade in the bowl. Cook the tempeh for 3 minutes, until browned on the bottom. Flip the tempeh, pour the rest of the marinade into the pan, and cook for an additional 2 minutes on the other side, until both sides are browned and the marinade has reduced and become a sticky glaze on the tempeh.

TO STORE: Refrigerate in an airtight container for up to 4 days.

TO REHEAT: Warm in a frying pan over low heat until the desired temperature is reached.

VARIATION: Peanut Skillet Tempeh. Omit the vinaigrette. Whisk the maple syrup with ¼ cup (60ml) Pantry Peanut Sauce (page 243) and 2 tablespoons lime juice. Marinate as directed above, then cook the tempeh over medium-low heat instead of medium.

NUTRITION:
239 calories | **18.2g** fat | **10.2g** protein | **11.2g** total carbs | **2.5g** sugar alcohols | **2.6g** net carbs

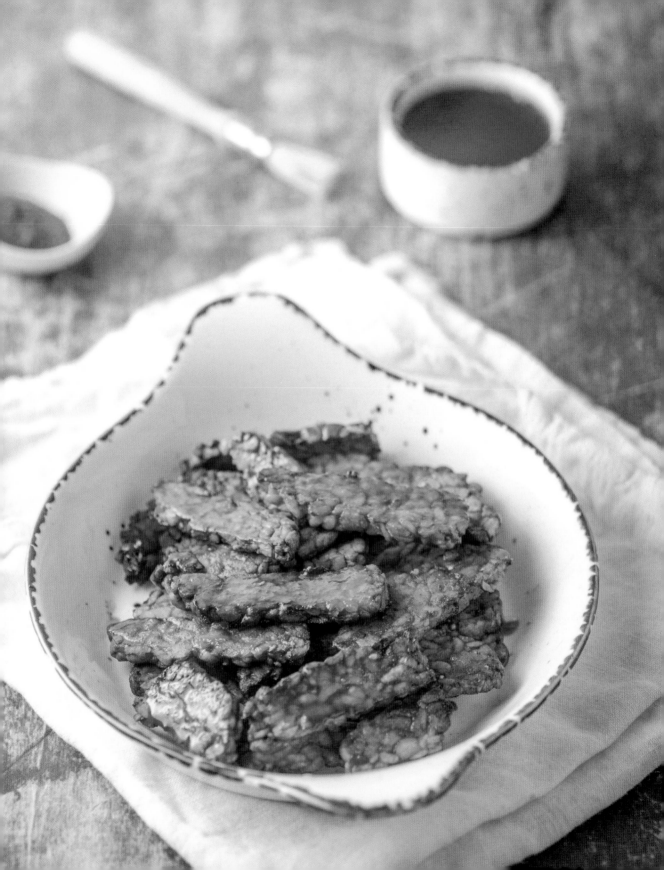

Mushroom "Meatballs"

YIELD: 3 servings

PREP TIME: 10 minutes

COOK TIME: 25 minutes

Yes, you can buy premade mock meatballs at the store, but I like making my own food whenever possible. One benefit is that you can control the quality of the ingredients. You can also control the flavor and texture. I like to play around with how finely I chop the mushrooms for these "meatballs," leaving some slightly larger bits for a meatier texture instead of blending them until they're completely smooth.

1 tablespoon extra-virgin olive oil

8 ounces (225g) button or cremini mushrooms, sliced

½ teaspoon dried oregano leaves

1 teaspoon dehydrated onion flakes

¼ teaspoon salt

¼ cup (40g) hulled hemp seeds

¼ cup (64g) tahini

1 tablespoon psyllium husks

TO STORE: Refrigerate in an airtight container for up to 4 days.

TO REHEAT: Warm in a preheated 300°F (150°C) oven for about 5 minutes, until warmed through.

- Preheat the oven to 350°F (177°C) and line a rimmed baking sheet with parchment paper.

- Heat the oil in a medium frying pan over medium heat. Add the mushrooms, oregano, onion flakes, and salt and cook, stirring occasionally, until the mushrooms are completely softened, about 5 minutes. Remove the pan from the heat and let cool for about 5 minutes.

- While the mushrooms are cooling, blend the hemp seeds in a food processor until finely ground.

- Add the cooled mushrooms, tahini, and psyllium husks to the food processor and continue blending until a "dough" forms. You can continue blending until it is smooth, but I like to leave larger bits of mushroom intact. Let the mixture sit for 5 minutes to allow the psyllium to gel.

- Form the mushroom mixture into nine equal-sized balls, about 1½ tablespoons each. Place the balls on the lined baking sheet and bake for 20 minutes, or until the balls are firm and starting to brown on the outside.

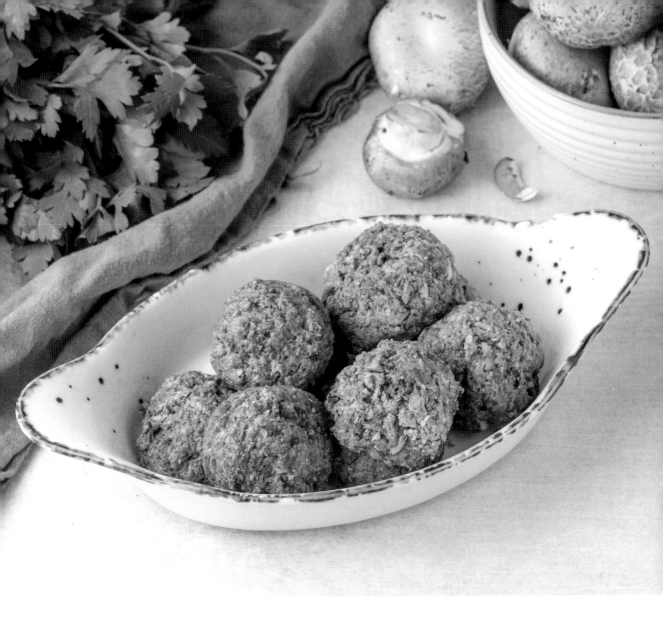

VARIATIONS:

Garlic Sesame "Meatballs." **Replace the olive oil with toasted sesame oil. Replace the oregano and onion flakes with 1 tablespoon minced garlic. Stir 2 tablespoons sesame seeds into the mushroom mixture before forming into meatballs.**

Cumin Spice "Meatballs." **Replace the oregano with 1 tablespoon dried parsley, 1 teaspoon ground cumin, ¾ teaspoon smoked paprika, and ¼ teaspoon ground cinnamon.**

NUTRITION:
284 calories | **22.2g** fat | **12.6g** protein | **11.7g** total carbs | **5.5g** net carbs

Vegan Feta

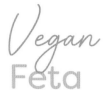

YIELD: about 1 pound (2 ounces/ 60g per serving)

PREP TIME: 5 minutes, plus 8 hours to set up

Yes, you can buy vegan versions of feta, but making your own gives you about three times the yield for half the cost, and the homemade version is much higher in protein. If you can't tolerate soy, you can use hemp tofu in place of regular tofu and a chickpea miso paste.

While the miso paste isn't necessary for this recipe to work, it adds a fermented tangy flavor to this faux feta, bringing it closer in taste to the real thing.

12 ounces (340g) extra-firm tofu, drained and pressed

½ cup (120ml) melted coconut oil

2 tablespoons nutritional yeast

1 tablespoon apple cider vinegar

1 teaspoon white miso (optional)

½ teaspoon salt

- Line a 9 by 5-inch (23 by 12.75-cm) loaf pan with parchment paper or cheesecloth.

- Blend the tofu, coconut oil, nutritional yeast, vinegar, miso (if using), and salt in a high-powered blender or food processor until completely smooth, scraping down the sides as needed, 1 to 2 minutes.

- Pour the mixture into the lined pan and refrigerate for 8 hours, until firm.

TO STORE: Refrigerate in an airtight container for up to a week, or freeze for up to a month.

NUTRITION:
169 calories | **15.6g** fat | **5.1g** protein | **2.2g** total carbs | **1.4g** net carbs

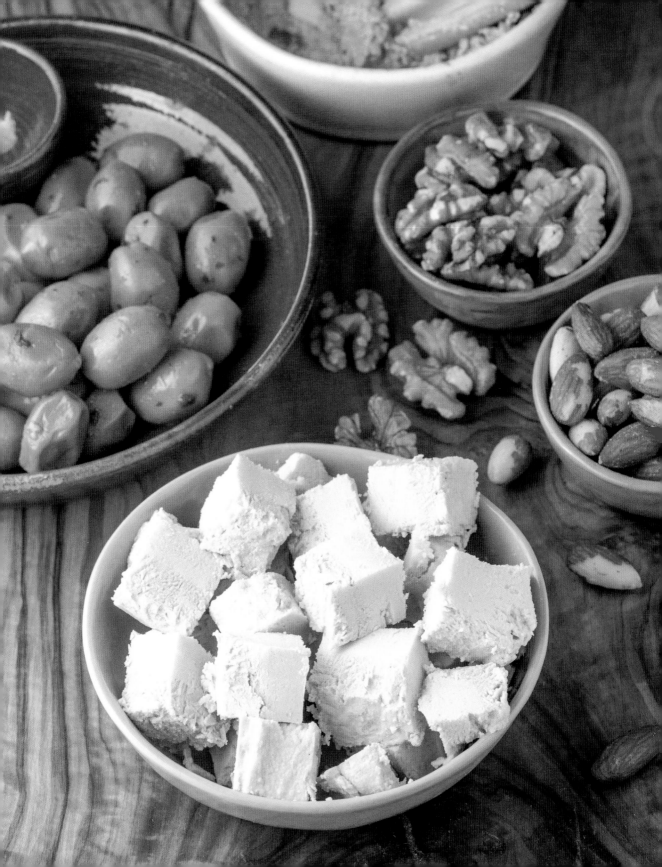

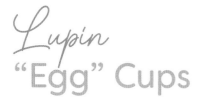

Lupin "Egg" Cups

YIELD: 6 servings

PREP TIME: 10 minutes

COOK TIME: 30 minutes

One of the requests I receive most often is to come up with soy-free vegan egg bites, which are usually made with tofu. While the texture of these isn't exactly the same as tofu egg cups, it's surprisingly close! If you want to add flavors, I recommend sticking with dried herbs and spices. I tried mixing in a lot of different ingredients, and fresh herbs and vegetables added too much moisture.

¼ **cup (30g) lupin flour**

¼ **cup (16g) nutritional yeast**

2 **tablespoons chickpea flour**

1½ **teaspoons psyllium husks**

1 **teaspoon baking powder**

¼ **teaspoon black salt (kala namak) or other salt of choice (see Notes)**

¾ **cup (180ml) pea milk or other nondairy milk of choice (see Notes)**

2 **tablespoons extra-virgin olive oil, plus extra for greasing the pan**

- Preheat the oven to 350°F (177°C) and lightly grease six wells of a standard silicone or nonstick muffin pan with olive oil.

- In a medium bowl, whisk together the lupin flour, nutritional yeast, chickpea flour, psyllium husks, baking powder, and salt until thoroughly combined. Slowly whisk in the milk and oil and continue whisking until just combined. Let the batter sit for 5 minutes, until the psyllium gels and the batter thickens. The batter should be just too thick to pour.

- Divide the batter evenly among the prepared muffin cups and bake for 30 minutes, or until firm to the touch.

- Let cool in the pan for at least 10 minutes, until the egg cups are set. Carefully remove from the pan and serve.

TO STORE: Refrigerate in an airtight container for up to 5 days, or freeze for up to a month.

TO REHEAT: Warm in a preheated 300°F (150°C) oven for about 5 minutes, until warmed through.

VARIATION: Garlic-Chive "Egg" Cups. Whisk in 1 tablespoon dried chives and ½ teaspoon granulated garlic with the dry ingredients.

NOTES: Kala namak is a salt from South Asia that is rich in sulfur and imparts an eggy taste and smell. I usually get mine from the Indian food section of the grocery store. If you can't find kala namak (or don't want to buy a specialty ingredient for just one recipe, which is totally understandable), you can use any salt you like. Truffle salt works nicely here, but plain salt is fine, too.

I use pea milk in this recipe because of the higher protein content. The brand I typically buy is Ripple, though I have also successfully used NotMilk. Soy milk has similar macros and is a great alternative if you can tolerate soy. If beans don't sit well with you, any nondairy milk will work here, but the protein content will be lower.

NUTRITION:
81 calories | **5.6g** fat | **4.6g** protein | **4.6g** total carbs | **1.8g** net carbs

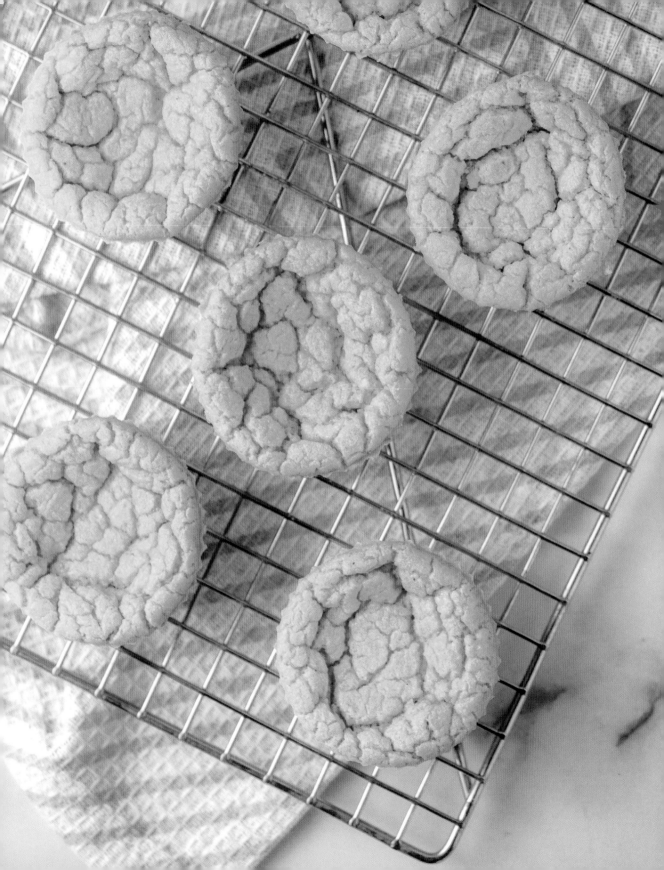

Super Savory
Instant Pot Pulled Pork Shoulder

YIELD: 8 servings

PREP TIME: 10 minutes

COOK TIME: 80 minutes

This is the tender and succulent pulled pork that you dream of! Pair it with Green Goddess Bowls (page 162) or Sesame-Garlic Kale (page 212) for an amazing dinner. In the variation below, sambal oelek, an Indonesian chile paste, brings a bright heat to the pork that will make your taste buds jump for joy!

1 (5-pound/2.25-kg) bone-in pork shoulder

1 tablespoon salt

1½ teaspoons smoked paprika

1 teaspoon onion powder

1 teaspoon ground black pepper

1 teaspoon dried parsley

1 tablespoon extra-virgin olive oil or avocado oil

1½ cups (355ml) chicken broth

2 teaspoons low-sodium tamari

TO STORE: Refrigerate the meat and desired amount of juices in an airtight container for up to 3 days, or freeze for up to 3 months. Freeze it in individual serving containers for a quick weeknight protein!

VARIATION: Spicy Citrus Sambal Pulled Pork Shoulder. Add 1 tablespoon sambal oelek, an additional 1 tablespoon tamari, 1 tablespoon lime juice, 1 tablespoon unseasoned rice vinegar, and 1 tablespoon grated fresh ginger to the Instant Pot when adding the broth before pressure cooking.

- Blot the pork shoulder dry with paper towels.

- In a small bowl, combine the salt, paprika, onion powder, pepper, and parsley. Rub the mixture all over the pork.

- Turn an Instant Pot to the "sauté" function. Add the oil to the pot when it's preheated.

- Gently place the seasoned pork shoulder in the Instant Pot. Sear for 3 minutes per side, then remove to a plate.

- Pour the chicken broth, tamari, and any accumulated meat juices from the plate into the pot. Using a wooden spoon, stir up all of the browned bits on the bottom.

- Return the pork to the pot. Cover and turn the pressure valve to "sealing."

- Turn the Instant Pot to the "manual" function and pressure cook on high for 80 minutes. Let the pressure release naturally for 15 minutes, then turn the pressure valve from "sealing" to "venting" and manually release any remaining steam.

- Transfer the pork to a large meat cutting board or a large bowl to collect the flavorful juices. Remove the meat from the bone and shred with two forks.

NUTRITION:
425 calories | **26.5g** fat | **43.3g** protein | **0.9g** total carbs | **0.6g** net carbs

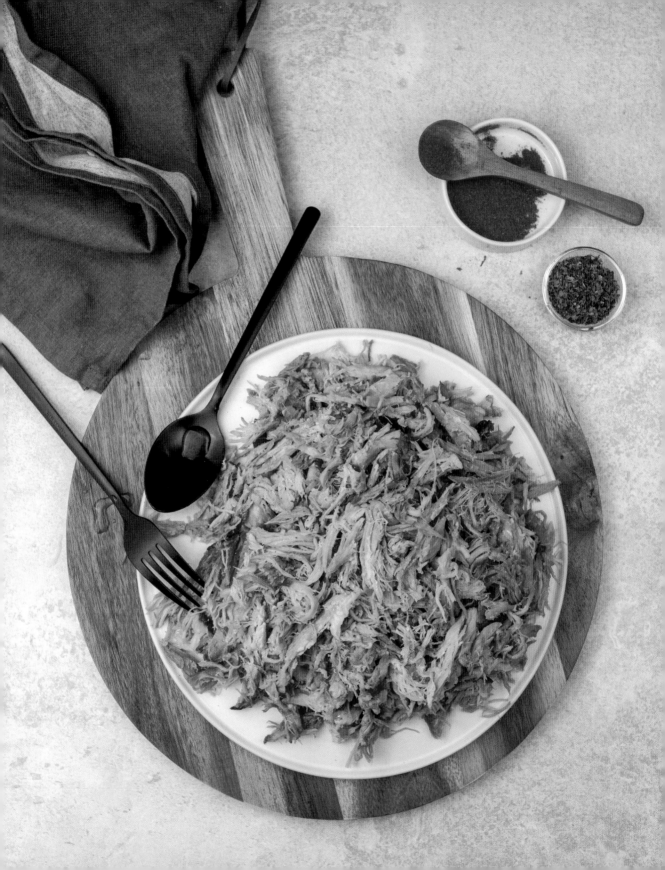

Grilled
Chicken Mole

YIELD: 4 servings

PREP TIME: 15 minutes, plus 20 minutes to soak peppers and 1 hour to marinate chicken

COOK TIME: 90 minutes

This spicy and complexly flavored mole brings a whole world of deliciousness to chicken thighs. Mole-marinated chicken chars up beautifully on the grill, making it the perfect food for a night under the stars. It would be fantastic charred up on a grill pan in the kitchen, too! Shred it and use it instead of the plant-based protein in the Empanada-Inspired Collard Wraps (page 150), or use half of each! This chicken also pairs well with Rainbow Veggie Pilaf (page 214).

MOLE

2 medium plum tomatoes, halved

1 tablespoon extra-virgin olive oil

½ teaspoon salt

½ teaspoon ground black pepper

3 dried ancho chiles

1 dried guajillo chile

2 tablespoons raw almonds

2 cups (475ml) chicken broth

1 tablespoon apple cider vinegar

1 tablespoon tomato paste

2 teaspoons dried oregano leaves

2 teaspoons ground cumin

¾ teaspoon smoked paprika

2 teaspoons liquid stevia

1 bay leaf

4 bone-in, skin-on chicken thighs (about 1½ pounds/680g)

- Preheat the oven to 400°F (204°C). Line a rimmed baking sheet with parchment paper.

- Place the tomatoes on the lined baking sheet, drizzle with the oil, and season with the salt and pepper. Bake for 20 minutes, or until lightly caramelized. When done, remove from the oven, let cool, and coarsely chop.

- While the tomatoes are baking, prepare the chiles: Toast the ancho and guajillo chiles in a large, dry frying pan over medium heat until fragrant, 3 to 4 minutes. Transfer the peppers to a plate and let cool. When cool, remove the seeds and stems and coarsely chop the peppers.

- Place the chopped peppers in a medium bowl and cover with boiling water. Cover the bowl with plastic wrap or a tight-fitting cover and let sit for 20 minutes, or until softened. When done, remove the peppers from the water; discard the soaking liquid.

- In the same frying pan, toast the almonds over medium-low heat, stirring often, until fragrant, 3 to 4 minutes. Remove the nuts from the pan and let cool. When cool, coarsely chop.

- Place the tomatoes, chiles, and almonds in a blender with the broth, vinegar, tomato paste, oregano, cumin, and paprika and process until smooth.

TO STORE: Shredded chicken in mole sauce can be portioned into individual containers (alternatively, you can store the shredded chicken and the mole in separate containers) and refrigerated for up to 3 days or frozen for up to 3 months.

VARIATION: Lemon Pepper Grilled Chicken Mole. Brush the chicken with avocado oil and season with salt and lemon pepper. Grill the chicken until cooked through, then shred the chicken and toss with the mole.

- Pour the sauce into a medium Dutch oven with the stevia and bay leaf. Bring to a gentle boil over medium heat. Reduce the heat to medium-low and simmer until the sauce is thick enough to coat the back of a spoon, 30 to 40 minutes. Let the mole cool completely.

- Place the chicken in a large resealable plastic bag. Cover with 1½ cups of the cooled mole and seal the bag. Work the bag with your hands so that the chicken is completely covered. Marinate in the refrigerator for 1 hour. Keep the remaining 1 cup of mole covered and refrigerated.

- Preheat a grill to medium-high heat.

- Remove the chicken from the mole marinade; discard the leftover marinade. Grease the grill grates. Place the thighs skin side down on the grill and cook with the lid closed until charred, about 10 minutes.

- Flip the chicken and reduce the grill heat to medium. Continue cooking until the meat in the thickest part of a thigh registers 165°F (74°C), 20 to 25 minutes.

- Just before serving, gently warm the reserved mole.

- Serve the chicken thighs with the mole spooned over the top, or remove the chicken from the bone, shred it with two forks, and toss with the mole.

NUTRITION:
394 calories | **28.5g** fat | **25.9g** protein | **8.3g** total carbs | **5.6g** net carbs

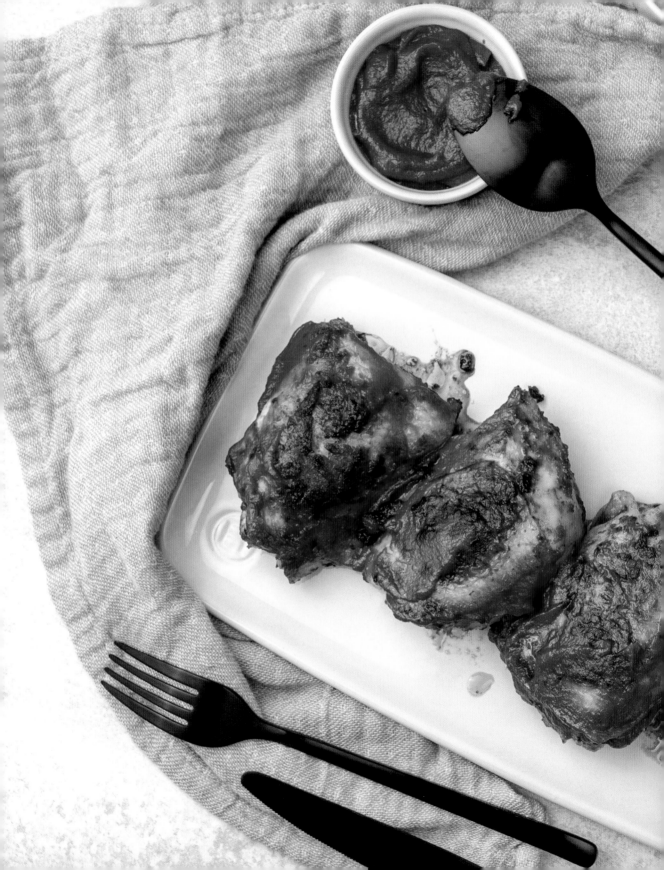

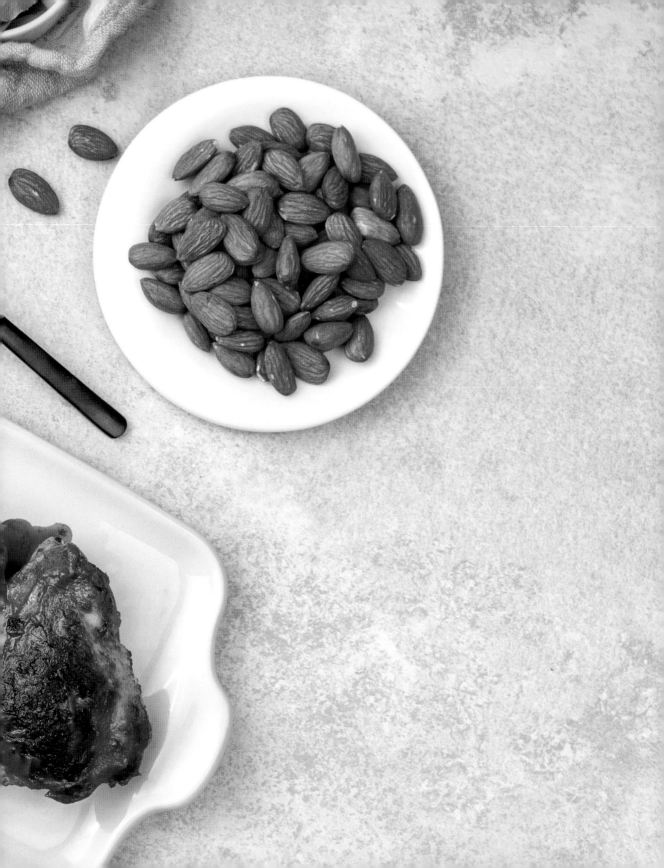

Keto Meatballs with Pine Nuts

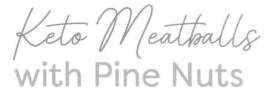

YIELD: 4 servings

PREP TIME: 10 minutes

COOK TIME: 15 minutes

Pine nuts give these savory meatballs a boost of flavor and good fat. The meatballs are the perfect protein accompaniment to Chimichurri Roasted Celeriac (page 222) or Harissa Roasted Carrots (page 218) for a scrumptious weeknight meal, or serve them as a light bite with Walnut Dressing (page 247) or Pistachio Parsley Pesto (page 246). And if you'd like to give them an amazing North African or Greek flair, there are a couple of variations below.

1 pound (454g) 80/20 ground beef

1 medium celery stalk, grated

1 tablespoon finely chopped pine nuts

2 teaspoons grated onion

1 teaspoon lemon pepper

½ teaspoon salt

1 large egg

- Preheat the oven to 425°F (218°C). Line a rimmed baking sheet with parchment paper.

- Place all of the ingredients in a large bowl. Lightly work the mixture until the ingredients are fully incorporated.

- Shape into 1½-inch (3.8-cm) balls and place them on the prepared baking sheet about 1 inch (2.5cm) apart.

- Bake for 12 to 15 minutes, or until cooked through (a meat thermometer should read 165°F [74°C] when inserted in a meatball).

TO STORE: Refrigerate in an airtight container for up to 2 days. Or, to freeze, place the meatballs on a rimmed baking sheet lined with parchment paper. Flash-freeze for 30 minutes, or until completely frozen. Store between layers of wax paper in a large, sturdy freezer container.

TO REHEAT: Warm the meatballs in a preheated 325°F (163°C) oven for 8 to 10 minutes, until warmed through.

VARIATIONS:

North African–Inspired Keto Meatballs. **Add 2 teaspoons ras el hanout to the meatball mixture. It adds an amazing warmth and depth of flavor to the meatballs that will keep you reaching for that magical spice blend over and over again! These would pair beautifully with Moroccan-Inspired Butternut Squash Stew (page 142), but, to keep the macros keto, omit the lupini beans from the stew.**

Greek-Inspired Keto Meatballs. **Add 2 tablespoons crumbled sheep's milk feta or Vegan Feta (page 180), 2 tablespoons chopped fresh parsley, 1½ teaspoons grated lemon zest, and 1 teaspoon ground cumin to the meatball mixture.**

NUTRITION:

324 calories | **21g** fat | **30.6g** protein | **1.3g** total carbs | **0.8g** net carbs

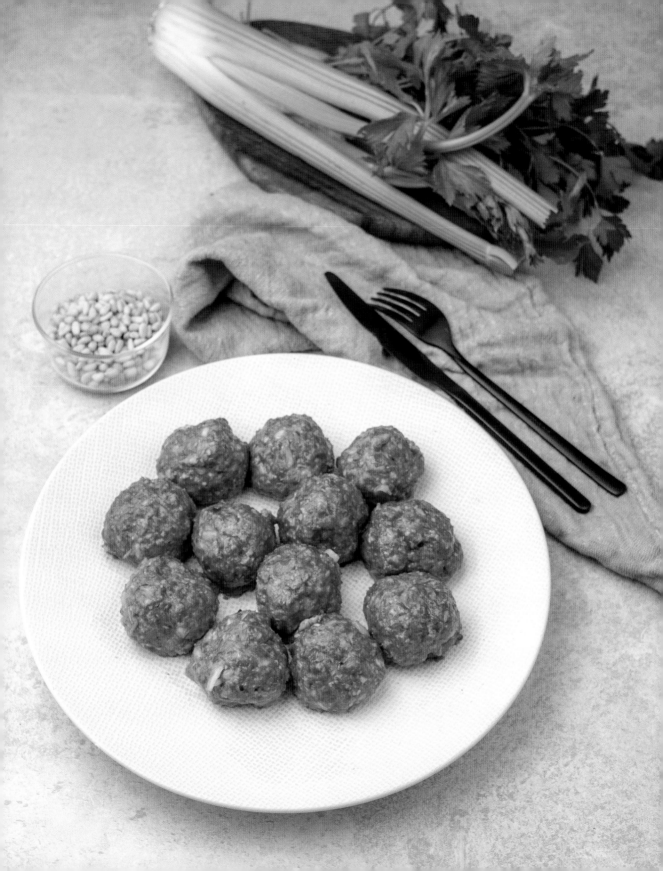

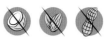

Grilled
Marinated Shrimp

YIELD: 4 servings

PREP TIME: 10 minutes

COOK TIME: 4 minutes

This shrimp couldn't be simpler to put together, and it packs a wallop of flavor. Serve it with the Pistachio Pesto Brussels Sprouts (page 224) and Sea Vegetable Salad (page 204) to round out the rainbow on your plate.

1 pound (454g) frozen 26/30 shrimp (peeled and deveined), thawed and patted dry

2 tablespoons extra-virgin olive oil, divided

2 teaspoons grated onion

2 teaspoons grated garlic

1½ teaspoons lemon pepper

1 teaspoon salt

- Preheat a grill pan or indoor grill to medium-high heat.

- While the grill pan or grill is preheating, place the shrimp in a large bowl and toss with 1 tablespoon of the oil, the grated onion and garlic, lemon pepper, and salt.

- Brush the grill pan ridges or grill grates with the remaining tablespoon of oil.

- Place the shrimp in the pan or on the grill and cook for 1 to 2 minutes. Flip and grill for an additional 1 to 2 minutes, until bright pink and cooked through. (You may have to cook the shrimp in batches so as not to crowd the grill pan.)

TO STORE: Refrigerate in an airtight container for up to 2 days.

TO REHEAT: Place the shrimp in a double boiler over simmering water and steam until warmed through.

VARIATION: Grilled Blackened Shrimp. Toss the shrimp with 2 tablespoons blackening seasoning along with the oil. This version would be amazing with Thai-Inspired Cauliflower Coconut Curry (page 144).

NUTRITION:
85 calories | **3.9g** fat | **13.3g** protein | **1g** total carbs | **0.9g** net carbs

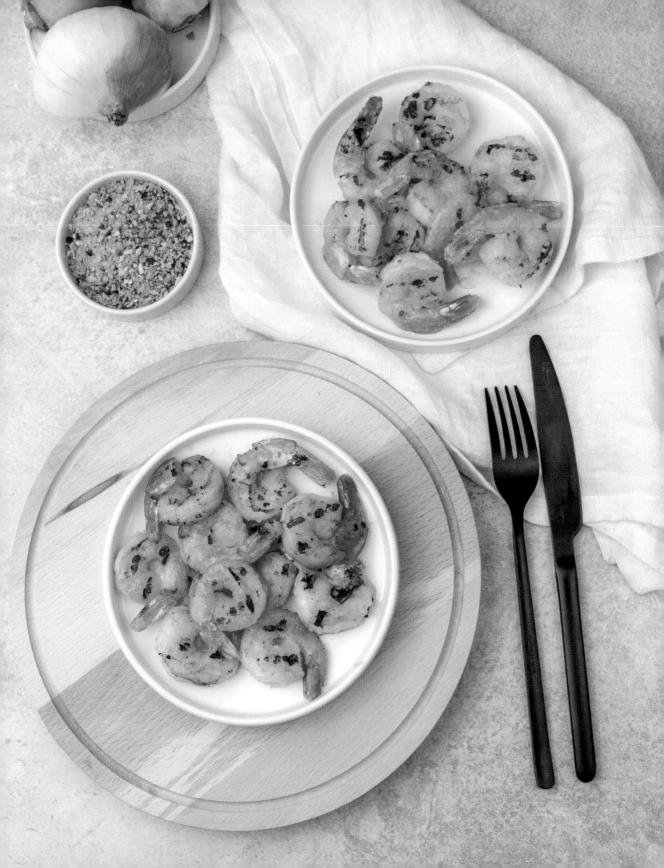

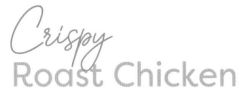

Crispy Roast Chicken

YIELD: 8 servings

PREP TIME: 15 minutes

COOK TIME: 70 minutes

If you're looking for a classic roast chicken, this is it! However, this is no ordinary roast chicken, because the high heat makes the skin beautifully crispy. Served with a side dish (see Chapter 4), this recipe is perfect for an evening meal for four, or you can freeze half of the chicken to have the base of a future weeknight meal ready to roll. Once shredded, this simply seasoned, versatile roast chicken can serve as a protein topper for just about any savory recipe in this book, from soups and salads to entrées and sides.

1 (3½-pound/1.5-kg) whole chicken

1 teaspoon salt

1 teaspoon lemon pepper

2 tablespoons extra-virgin olive oil

1 large lemon, quartered

4 sprigs fresh parsley

1 clove garlic, coarsely chopped

TO STORE: Refrigerate in an airtight container for up to 3 days.

TO REHEAT: Place the chicken pieces in an oven-safe container with a little bit of chicken broth to keep the meat moist. Cover and warm in a preheated 350°F (177°C) oven for 10 minutes. Remove the cover and cook for 2 minutes longer to recrisp the skin. To reheat shredded chicken, simply stir in a little bit of chicken broth to restore moisture and bake, covered, for 8 to 10 minutes.

- Preheat the oven to 425°F (218°C). Have on hand a roasting pan fitted with a roasting rack.

- Remove the giblets from the chicken cavity. Blot the chicken dry inside and out with paper towels. Season the chicken inside and out with the salt and lemon pepper. Tie the legs together with kitchen twine. Brush the chicken all over with the oil.

- Insert the lemon quarters, parsley, and garlic into the chicken cavity. Set the chicken on the roasting rack in the roasting pan.

- Roast until the chicken registers 165°F (74°C) on a meat thermometer inserted into the thickest part of a thigh, 60 to 70 minutes.

- Place the chicken on a large cutting board and let rest, uncovered, for 10 minutes.

- Carve and serve immediately, or let cool, remove the skin and meat from the bones, and shred the chicken.

VARIATION: Crispy Ras el Hanout Roast Chicken. Season the chicken inside and out with a mixture of 1 tablespoon ras el hanout and 1 teaspoon each salt and unsalted lemon pepper before roasting. Alternatively, season the shredded cooked chicken with ras el hanout to taste.

NUTRITION:
223 calories | **14.2g** fat | **21.9g** protein | **0.8g** total carbs | **0.2g** net carbs

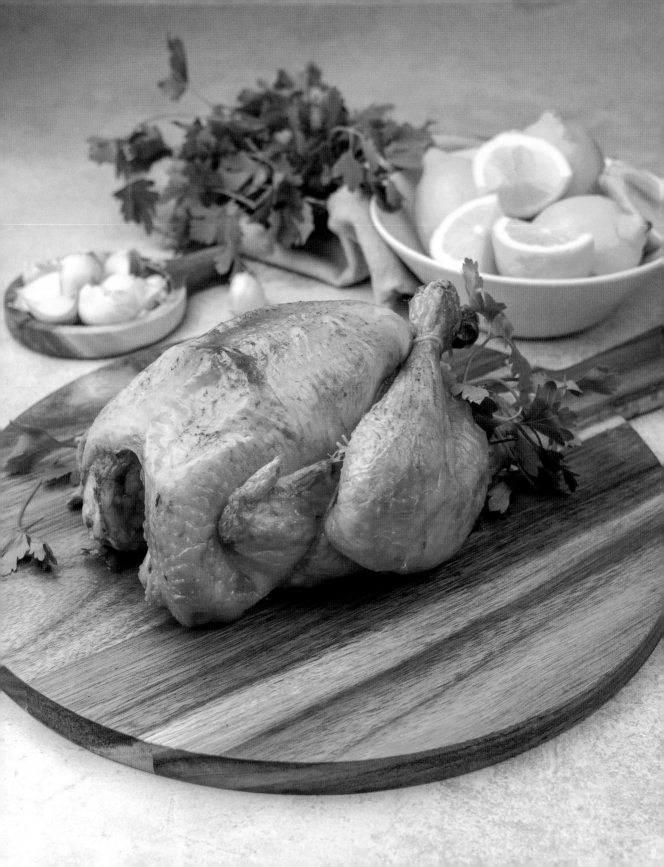

Marinated Pan-Fried Rib Eye

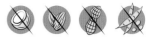

YIELD: 4 servings

PREP TIME: 2 minutes, plus 45 minutes to marinate

COOK TIME: 8 minutes

This rib eye is succulent, buttery, and ultra-savory. Serve it with Balsamic Beets & Greens (page 216) along with Dark Chocolate Truffles (page 252) to round out an amazing date-night meal!

3 tablespoons extra-virgin olive oil, divided

1 clove garlic, minced

1 teaspoon kosher salt

1 teaspoon ground black pepper

1 (1¼- to 1½-pound/560- to 680-g) boneless grass-fed rib-eye steak, approximately 1 inch (2.5cm) thick

1 tablespoon grass-fed ghee

1 tablespoon grass-fed butter

2 teaspoons fresh thyme leaves

TO STORE: Refrigerate in an airtight container for up to 3 days.

TO REHEAT: Place in an oven-safe container with a little of the pan juices to keep the meat moist. Cover and warm in a preheated 350°F (177°C) oven for 10 to 12 minutes, until warmed through.

VARIATION: *Tamari-Mustard Rib Eye.* Add 1 tablespoon low-sodium tamari and 2 teaspoons Dijon mustard to the marinade and reduce the salt to ½ teaspoon.

- Put 2 tablespoons of the oil, the garlic, salt, and pepper in a small bowl; whisk until well combined.

- Place the rib eye in a large glass container and rub the marinade on all sides of it. Cover with plastic wrap and refrigerate for 20 minutes, flipping the steak after 10 minutes. Remove from the refrigerator and let sit at room temperature for 20 minutes.

- Remove the rib eye from the marinade and blot it dry with paper towels. Discard any remaining marinade.

- Heat the ghee and the remaining tablespoon of oil in a large cast-iron skillet over medium heat. When the ghee has melted and the fats are hot but not smoking, add the rib eye to the pan.

- Cook for 4 minutes. Flip and cook for an additional 4 minutes. Add the butter and thyme; once the butter has melted, spoon the fat in the skillet over the steak.

- At this point, the steak should be cooked to medium-rare doneness. (A meat thermometer inserted in the center should read 125°F [52°C] to allow for residual-heat cooking when resting, giving a final temperature of 135°F [57°C].) Depending on the temperature you're looking for, you may need to flip it once more and cook it for 2 minutes longer. For the best flavor and texture, I don't recommend cooking it beyond medium doneness: 135°F (57°C) in the pan, 145°F (63°C) after resting.

- Place the steak on a cutting board and tent loosely with foil. Let it rest for 10 minutes before serving with the pan juices.

NUTRITION:
518 calories | **44.7g** fat | **29.2g** protein | **0.7g** total carbs | **0.5g** net carbs

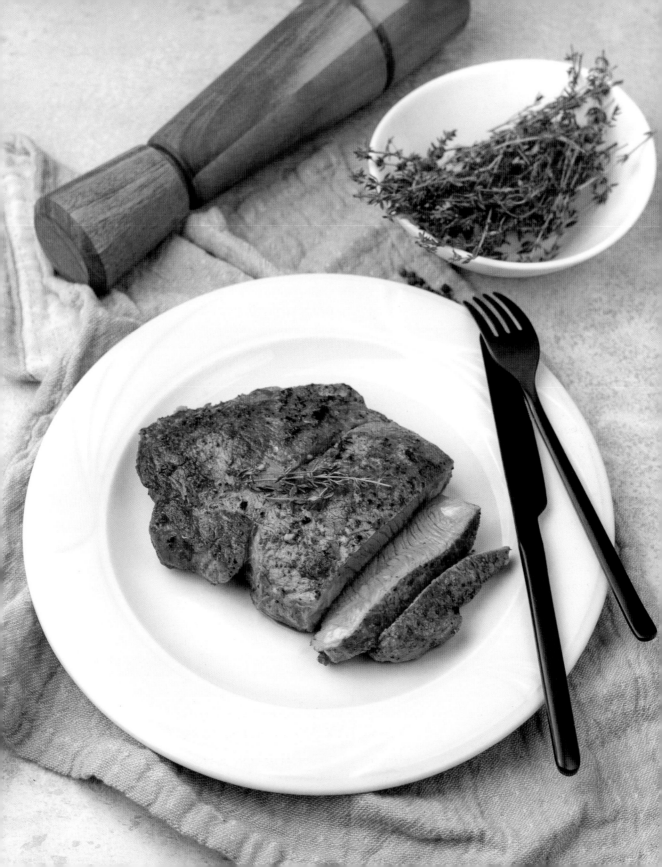

Succulent Flank Steak

YIELD: 4 servings

PREP TIME: 2 minutes plus 30 minutes to marinate

COOK TIME: 8 minutes

This steak is the perfect vehicle for a wide array of sauces or for use as a salad topper. Try serving a few slices atop Waldorf Kale Salad (page 132), a big plate of Cabbage & Kale Hash (page 100), or Mushroom Stroganoff (page 146)! It's also great with Chimichurri Roasted Celeriac (page 222).

The best classic sauce to serve this steak with is the chimichurri on page 242. While you can always choose to serve chimichurri alongside of flank steak as a condiment, another option is to slice the steak as it sits in a pool of chimichurri; the meat juices meld into the chimichurri, forming a super delicious sauce! (See the variation below.)

3 tablespoons extra-virgin olive oil, divided

1 clove garlic, coarsely chopped

1 teaspoon coarse sea salt, divided

1 teaspoon lemon pepper, divided

1½ pounds (680g) grass-fed flank steak

1 teaspoon dried parsley

1 teaspoon garlic powder

1 teaspoon onion powder

1 teaspoon smoked paprika

1 tablespoon grass-fed ghee

- Put 2 tablespoons of the oil, the garlic, ½ teaspoon of the salt, and ½ teaspoon of the lemon pepper in a small bowl; whisk until well combined.

- Place the steak in a glass container and rub the marinade on all sides of it. Let sit for 30 minutes at room temperature. Flip once after 15 minutes.

- Remove the steak from the marinade and blot it dry with paper towels. Discard any remaining marinade.

- In a small bowl, whisk together the parsley, garlic powder, onion powder, paprika, remaining ½ teaspoon of salt, and remaining ½ teaspoon of lemon pepper. Rub both sides of the steak with the seasoning mix.

- Heat the ghee and remaining tablespoon of oil in a large cast-iron skillet over medium heat. When the fats are hot but not smoking, add the steak to the pan. Sear for 2 minutes, flip, and sear for another 2 minutes. Repeat once more for a total of 8 minutes of cooking time.

- At this point, the steak should be cooked to medium-rare doneness. (A meat thermometer inserted in the center should

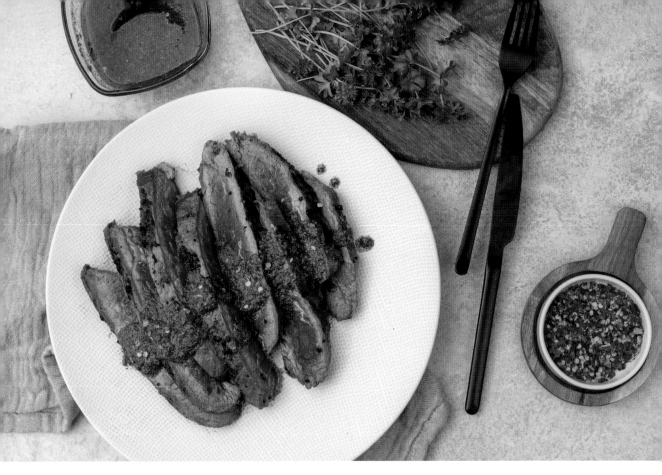

TO STORE: Refrigerate in an airtight container for up to 3 days.

TO REHEAT: Place in an oven-safe container with some of the pan juices to keep the meat moist. Cover and bake in a preheated 350°F (177°C) oven for about 10 minutes, until warmed through.

read 125°F [52°C] to allow for residual-heat cooking when resting, giving a final temperature of 135°F [57°C].) For the best flavor and texture, I don't recommend cooking it beyond medium doneness: 135°F (57°C) in the pan, 145°F (63°C) after resting.

- Tent the steak loosely with foil to allow it to finish cooking and the juices to redistribute; let rest for 10 minutes. To serve, slice thinly across the grain.

VARIATION: Chimichurri Flank Steak. Spread about 1 cup Chimichurri (page 242) on a large cutting board (preferably with grooves to catch the juices), in the approximate shape and size of the flank steak. When the steak is cooked, remove it from the skillet and place it directly on the sauce. Tent the steak loosely with foil and let rest for 10 minutes. Slice the steak thinly across the grain and transfer to a serving platter. Pour the sauce and meat juices left on the cutting board into a bowl, stir to combine, and serve with the steak.

NUTRITION:
379 calories | **23.3g** fat | **36.2g** protein | **1.5g** total carbs | **1.3g** net carbs

Oven-Roasted New York Strip Steak

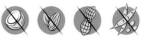

YIELD: 4 servings

PREP TIME: 1 minute, plus 30 minutes for steak to come to room temperature

COOK TIME: 10 minutes

Sometimes the simplest preparation just lets a steak shine. And when it comes to pairing this flavorful steak, well, look no further than Broccoli Tots (page 228) and Veggie Flatbreads (page 140).

1½ pounds (680g) boneless grass-fed New York strip steak, 1 inch (2.5cm) to 1¾ inches (4cm) thick

1 tablespoon extra-virgin olive oil

1 teaspoon coarse sea salt

1 teaspoon coarsely ground black pepper

TO STORE: Refrigerate in an airtight container for up to 3 days.

TO REHEAT: Place in a small baking dish with a little chicken or beef broth to keep it moist. Cover and warm in a preheated 350°F (177°C) oven for 10 minutes, or until warmed through.

- About 30 minutes before cooking, take the steak out of the refrigerator and set aside at room temperature.

- Place a large cast-iron skillet in a cold oven. Preheat the oven to 450°F (232°C).

- When the oven comes to temperature, brush the steak on both sides with the oil and season on both sides with the salt and pepper.

- Carefully remove the pan from the oven; it will be very hot! Do not turn off the oven.

- Place the steak in the hot pan and sear for 2 minutes without moving it. Then, using a pair of tongs, sear the edges of the steak.

- Flip the steak so that the seared side is up and carefully place the pan back into the oven. Roast for 3 to 5 minutes, or until it reaches 125°F (52°C) for medium-rare. If you prefer your steak at medium doneness, roast for another 2 to 3 minutes, or until it reaches 135°F (57°C).

- Remove the pan from the oven and place the steak on a cutting board. Tent loosely with foil and let rest for 10 minutes to allow it to finish cooking and the juices to redistribute.

NUTRITION:
411 calories | **29.2g** fat | **35g** protein | **0.4g** total carbs | **0.3g** net carbs

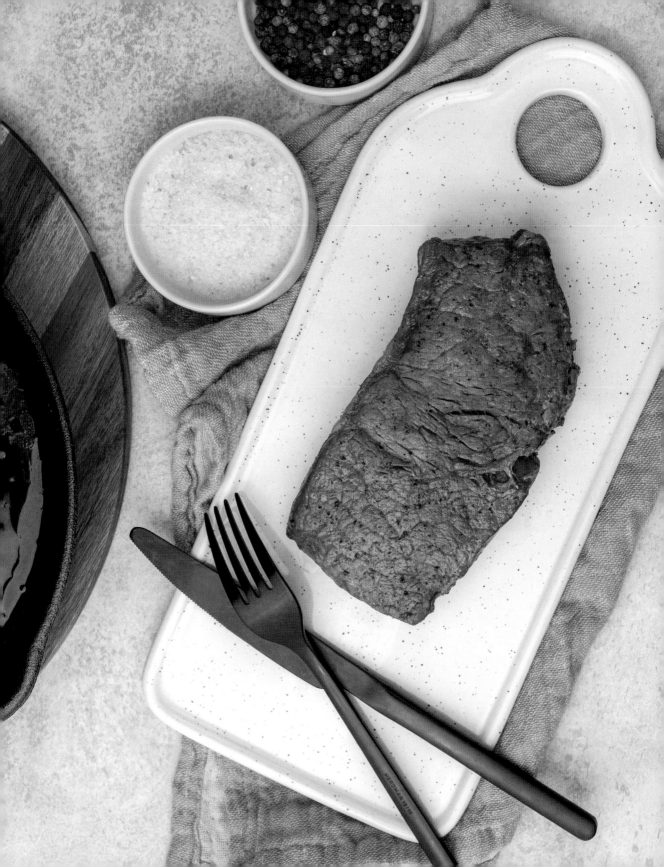

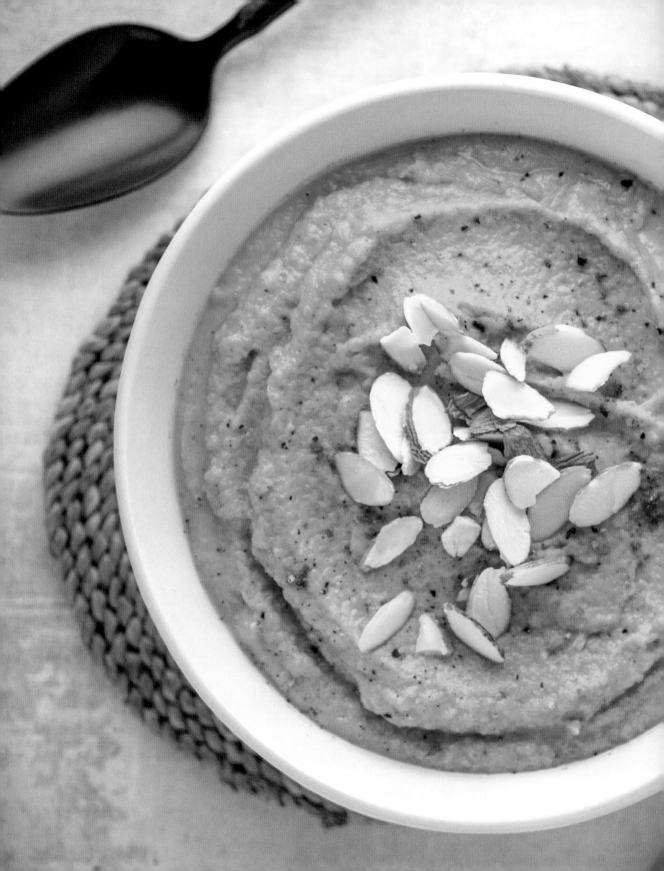

CHAPTER 4:

Side Dishes & Small Bites

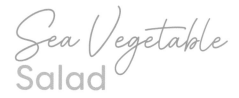

Sea Vegetable Salad

YIELD: 4 servings

PREP TIME: 10 minutes

Maybe I don't pay enough attention on social media, but I feel like there is a distinct lack of seaweed representation in most keto diets. While keto sushi-style rolls do pop up on my feed from time to time, I rarely see any other type of sea vegetable, and when I do, it is usually roasted nori snacks. I think we're missing out by not including more seaweed: not only is it delicious (and a rich source of iodine), but kelp noodles are nice and crunchy, which is hard to come by in keto foods. This keto seaweed salad, with two types of sea vegetables, makes a great side for the chili-lime variation of the Super Crispy Baked Tofu (page 172).

1 (12-ounce/340-g) package kelp noodles

5 sheets sushi nori

2 tablespoons low-sodium tamari

2 tablespoons toasted sesame oil

1 tablespoon unseasoned rice wine vinegar

2 tablespoons water

½ teaspoon crushed garlic

½ teaspoon grated fresh ginger

1 tablespoon sesame seeds

2 scallions (green parts only), sliced, for garnish

- Drain and rinse the kelp noodles, then place them in a medium bowl. Using a pair of kitchen shears, cut the noodles to break up the clumps and make them easier to mix.

- Using the shears or a very sharp knife, cut the nori sheets into ½-inch (1.25-cm) strips (see Note). Place the nori strips in the bowl with the kelp noodles.

- In a small bowl, whisk together the tamari, sesame oil, vinegar, water, garlic, and ginger and pour over the nori strips. As the nori and kelp absorb the liquid, they will soften and the nori will reduce in volume. Stir the seaweed until all of the liquid is absorbed and the seaweed is uniformly hydrated, 1 to 2 minutes.

- Stir in the sesame seeds and divide the salad among four serving bowls. Garnish with the scallions and enjoy!

NOTE: The nori sheets that I use have perforations, and I find it easiest to stack two or three sheets, fold them along those lines, and then cut that folded stack crosswise into strips.

TO STORE: Refrigerate in an airtight container for up to 4 days.

NUTRITION:
93 calories | **8.4g** fat | **3.1g** protein | **6.1g** total carbs | **1.9g** net carbs

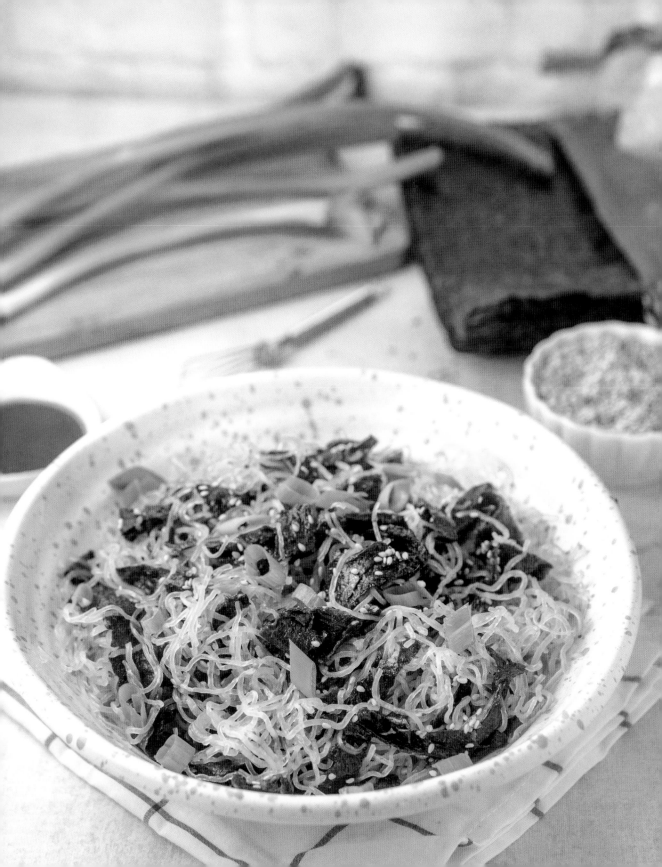

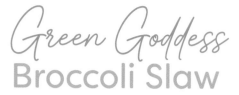

Green Goddess Broccoli Slaw

YIELD: 4 servings

PREP TIME: 5 minutes (not including time to make dressing)

This slaw has become my favorite side for a veggie burger on a hot summer day, which I realize is a pretty specific scenario, but is also pretty common for two-ish months of the year. There's something about green goddess dressing that is just so refreshing, and I love adding seeds to dishes for some textural interest.

If you have a difficult time digesting seeds, you can either replace them with your favorite chopped nuts or omit them entirely.

1 (12-ounce/340-g) package broccoli slaw (see Note)

¼ cup (30g) shelled pumpkin seeds (pepitas)

½ cup (120ml) Green Goddess Dressing (page 241)

2 scallions (green parts only), thinly sliced on the diagonal, for garnish

Red pepper flakes, for garnish (optional)

In a large bowl, mix together the broccoli slaw, pumpkin seeds, and dressing until the broccoli is well coated. Sprinkle the scallions on top to serve. Garnish with red pepper flakes, if desired.

NOTE: You can make your own broccoli slaw by using a mandoline slicer to cut a peeled broccoli stem into matchsticks. You can also make the slaw with thinly sliced cabbage instead.

TO STORE: Refrigerate in an airtight container for up to 3 days.

NUTRITION:
114 calories | **8.2g** fat | **4.5g** protein | **7.7g** total carbs | **3.4g** net carbs

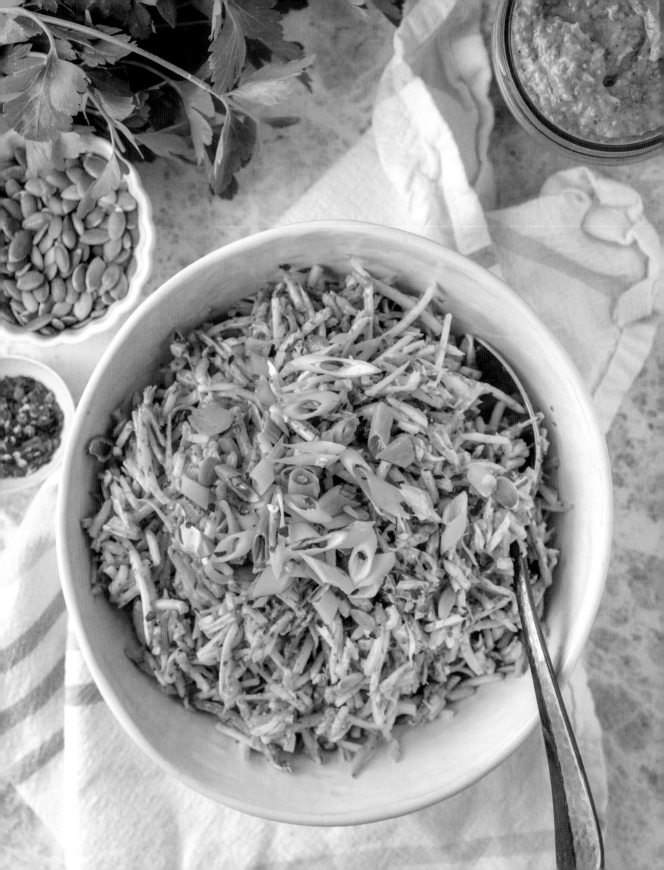

Greek-Inspired
Cucumber Boats

YIELD: 6 servings

PREP TIME: 10 minutes (not including time to make feta or dressing)

I'm a big fan of Kalamata olives and will pass up no opportunity to eat them. See also: feta (although the feta I've been eating for the last decade has been a dairy-free version). These cucumber boats are full of flavor, though they make for a pretty light and refreshing snack. If you can't find Persian (mini) cucumbers, you could slice a large cucumber into rounds and use the filling as a dip for them.

3 Persian cucumbers

2 ounces (60g) Vegan Feta (page 180) or sheep's milk feta

¼ cup (30g) pitted Kalamata olives

1 tablespoon minced red onions

1 tablespoon Sun-Dried Tomato Dressing (page 245)

1 teaspoon dried oregano leaves

SUGGESTED GARNISHES

Drizzle of Yogurt Dill Sauce (page 240)

Drizzle of Sun-Dried Tomato Dressing (page 245)

Red pepper flakes

Fresh ground black pepper

- Slice the cucumbers in half lengthwise, then scoop out and discard the seeds. Scoop out about half of the remaining flesh on each cucumber half, leaving a trench for the filling, and set the cucumber boats and scooped-out flesh aside.

- In a food processor, pulse the cucumber flesh, feta, olives, onions, dressing, and oregano until coarsely chopped and combined. Be careful not to overprocess the ingredients.

- Divide the mixture among the cucumber boats and garnish as desired.

TO STORE: Refrigerate in an airtight container for up to 2 days.

NUTRITION:
62 calories | **5.4g** fat | **1.4g** protein | **2.3g** total carbs | **1.5g** net carbs

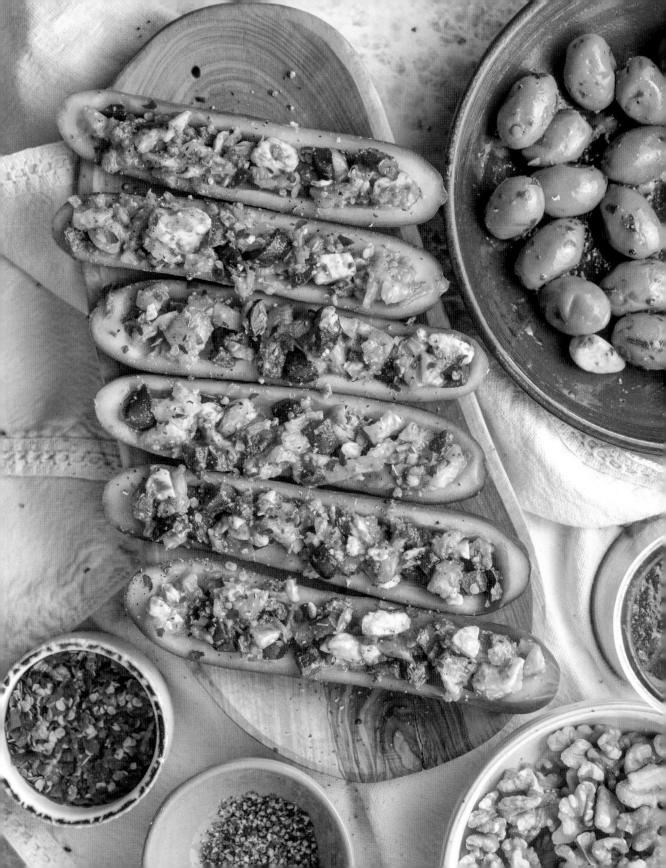

Raw Muhammara

YIELD: 1½ cups/360ml (¼ cup/ 60ml per serving)

PREP TIME: 8 minutes

Muhammara, a dip originating in Aleppo, Syria, is a blend of bell peppers, walnuts, and breadcrumbs that's flavored with cumin and pomegranate molasses. The traditional version is beyond delicious but needed some tweaking in order to be keto-friendly. I usually enjoy it with sliced vegetables or flax crackers.

Did you know that red bell peppers are a great source of vitamin C? They actually contain three times the vitamin C of oranges! Traditional muhammara is made with roasted peppers, but I like a raw version for a couple of reasons:

1) Vitamin C is heat-sensitive, so not cooking the peppers preserves their vitamin C content.

2) Sometimes I don't want to roast a pepper just to make a snack.

That being said, if you want to make a more traditional version of this dish, roast the pepper beforehand.

1 large red bell pepper (about 6 ounces/170g), cored, seeded, and sliced

1 cup (120g) roughly chopped raw walnuts

2 tablespoons extra-virgin olive oil

1 tablespoon lemon juice

2 cloves garlic, peeled

1 teaspoon ground cumin

½ teaspoon red pepper flakes

½ teaspoon salt

Smoked paprika, for sprinkling (optional)

Place the bell pepper, walnuts, oil, lemon juice, garlic, cumin, red pepper flakes, and salt in a food processor or high-powered blender and blend until smooth, 1 to 2 minutes. Transfer to a serving bowl and sprinkle with smoked paprika, if desired.

TO STORE: Refrigerate in an airtight container for up to 3 days.

MAKE IT MEDIUM-CARB: Add 2 teaspoons pomegranate molasses.

NUTRITION:
181 calories | **17.7g** fat | **3.4g** protein | **5g** total carbs | **3g** net carbs

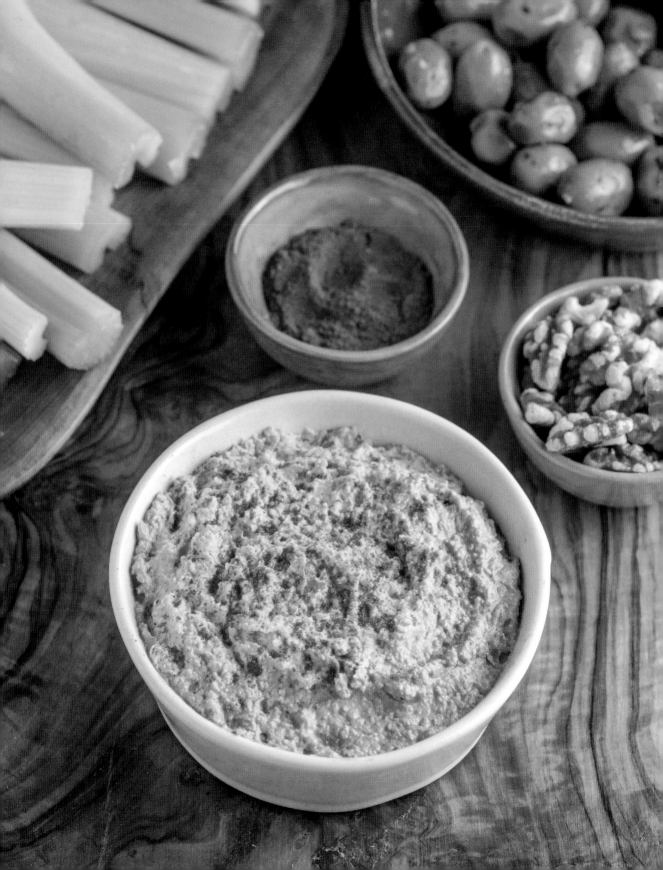

Sesame-Garlic Kale

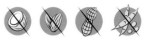

YIELD: 4 servings

PREP TIME: 8 minutes

COOK TIME: 12 minutes

Roasting is pretty much the easiest way to cook kale and, conveniently, I think it's also the best. Not only does the hot oven soften it and get rid of that tough texture, but the kale also gets nice and crispy along the edges. Sesame and garlic are such a simple combination of ingredients, but the flavor payoff far exceeds the effort!

I love this side so much that halfway through typing this headnote, I decided to make a batch for myself to go with lunch.

2 tablespoons toasted sesame oil

1 tablespoon minced garlic

¼ teaspoon salt

6 cups (125g) coarsely chopped kale (about 1 medium bunch)

1 scallion (green part only), thinly sliced on the diagonal

1 tablespoon sesame seeds

- Preheat the oven to 350°F (177°C) and line a rimmed baking sheet with parchment paper.

- In a large bowl, whisk together the oil, garlic, and salt. Add the kale and toss with the oil mixture until well coated. It's helpful to use your hands and really massage the oil into the leaves to soften them.

- Spread the kale in a thin layer on the lined baking sheet and roast for 12 minutes, until the edges of the kale are crispy.

- Transfer to a serving dish and sprinkle with the sliced scallion and sesame seeds.

TO STORE: Refrigerate in an airtight container for up to 3 days.

TO REHEAT: Warm in a small frying pan over low heat for about 5 minutes, until the desired temperature is reached.

NUTRITION:
90 calories | **8.7g** fat | **1.6g** protein | **2.5g** total carbs | **0.8g** net carbs

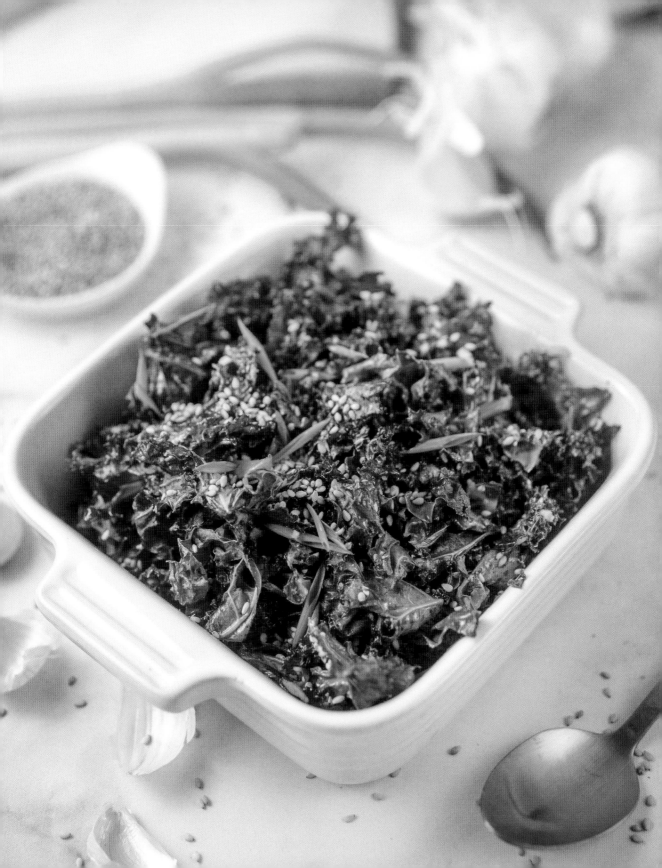

Rainbow Veggie Pilaf

YIELD: 6 servings

PREP TIME: 10 minutes

COOK TIME: 4 or 20 minutes, depending on method

Veggie rice is one of my favorite ways to use up the extra bits of vegetables that are hanging out in my fridge, reducing food waste. It only takes about a minute to turn broccoli stems, carrot chunks, and radishes into veggie rice. And, for convenience, I almost always have a bag of riced cauliflower in my freezer.

I grew up eating a lot of boxed pilaf. It just goes with everything. This is my keto interpretation, which can be made on the stovetop or in a pressure cooker. You can change the ratio of vegetables to match whatever you have on hand (which might just be two packages of riced cauliflower)—just so the total weight of the riced veggies is 24 ounces (680g). But keep in mind that this will change the macros.

1 (12-ounce/340-g) package frozen riced cauliflower

4 ounces (112g) riced broccoli stems

4 ounces (112g) riced carrots

4 ounces (112g) riced radishes

½ cup (60g) sunflower seeds

½ cup (120ml) vegetable broth

2 tablespoons extra-virgin olive oil

¾ teaspoon salt

½ teaspoon granulated garlic

Chopped fresh parsley, for garnish

- **To make on the stovetop:** Combine all of the ingredients except the parsley in a Dutch oven and cook over medium heat, stirring frequently, until the liquid has been absorbed and the vegetables are tender, about 20 minutes.

- **To make in a pressure cooker:** Combine all of the ingredients except the parsley in a pressure cooker, making sure to break up any large chunks of riced cauliflower, which tends to clump together. Secure the lid and cook on high pressure for 4 minutes. Let sit for about 5 minutes before carefully releasing the pressure manually.

- Stir and fluff the "rice" and garnish with fresh parsley to serve.

TO STORE: Refrigerate in an airtight container for up to 3 days.

TO REHEAT: Warm in a small frying pan over low heat for about 5 minutes, until the desired temperature is reached.

NUTRITION:
125 calories | **9.5g** fat | **3.8g** protein | 8.6g total carbs | **4.7g** net carbs

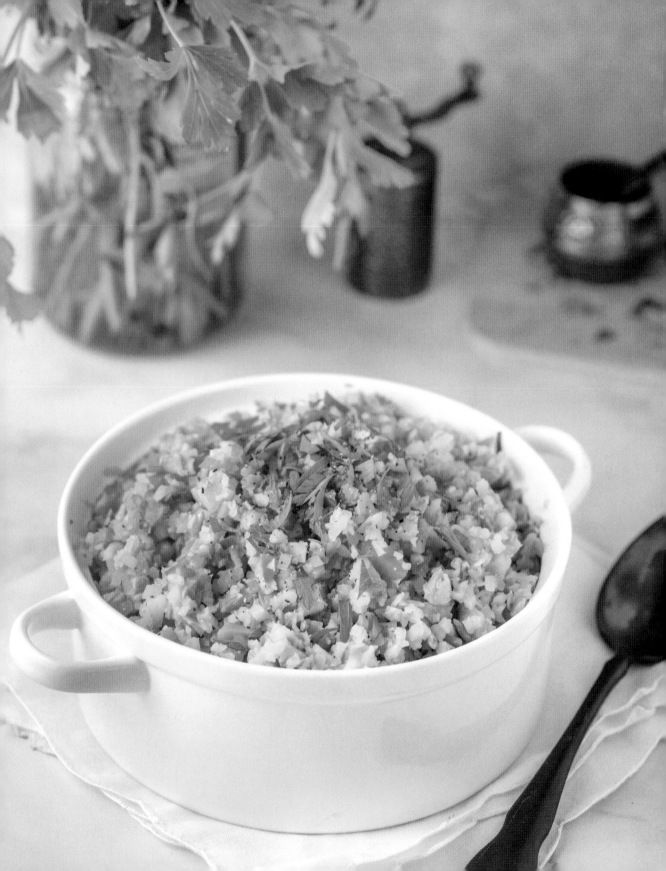

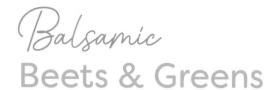

Balsamic Beets & Greens

YIELD: 4 servings

PREP TIME: 10 minutes (not including time to make vinaigrette)

COOK TIME: 35 minutes

Beets aren't the first vegetable that comes to mind when most people think of keto-friendly foods, but they're delicious and full of vitamins, minerals, and a slew of phytonutrients. So I think they're a worthwhile addition to any meal.

Similarly, beet greens are incredibly nutrient-dense—and quite tasty when roasted with some balsamic dressing! If your bunch of beets didn't come with the greens, you can use chard, collards, or kale instead.

1 small bunch beets with greens (about 9 ounces/255g)

4 tablespoons (60ml) Balsamic Vinaigrette (page 244), divided

TO STORE: Refrigerate in an airtight container for up to 3 days.

TO REHEAT: Warm in a small frying pan over low heat for about 5 minutes, until the desired temperature is reached.

MAKE IT MEDIUM-CARB: Double the quantity of beets and whisk 1 tablespoon maple syrup in with the vinaigrette before dividing.

- Preheat the oven to 375°F (190°C) and line a rimmed baking sheet with parchment paper.

- Cut the greens off the beets and set aside. Scrub the beets, peel them, if desired, and cut them in half crosswise. Cut the halves into quarters or eighths depending on size; the pieces should be about ½ inch (1.25 cm). Toss the beets in 2 tablespoons of the vinaigrette and spread out on the baking sheet. Roast for 25 minutes, until you can easily pierce the beets with a knife.

- While the beets are roasting, wash the greens and pat them dry with a clean kitchen towel. Roughly chop the greens (you should have about 2 cups/85g) and toss with the remaining 2 tablespoons of vinaigrette.

- After the beets have been roasting for 25 minutes, remove the baking sheet from the oven and push the beets to one side. Spread the beet greens in a thin layer on the other half of the baking sheet. Return the pan to the oven and roast for another 10 minutes, until the greens start to crisp up around the edges.

- Stir to mix the beets and greens together before serving.

NUTRITION:
117 calories | **10.2g** fat | **1.2g** protein | **5.8g** total carbs | **3.8g** net carbs

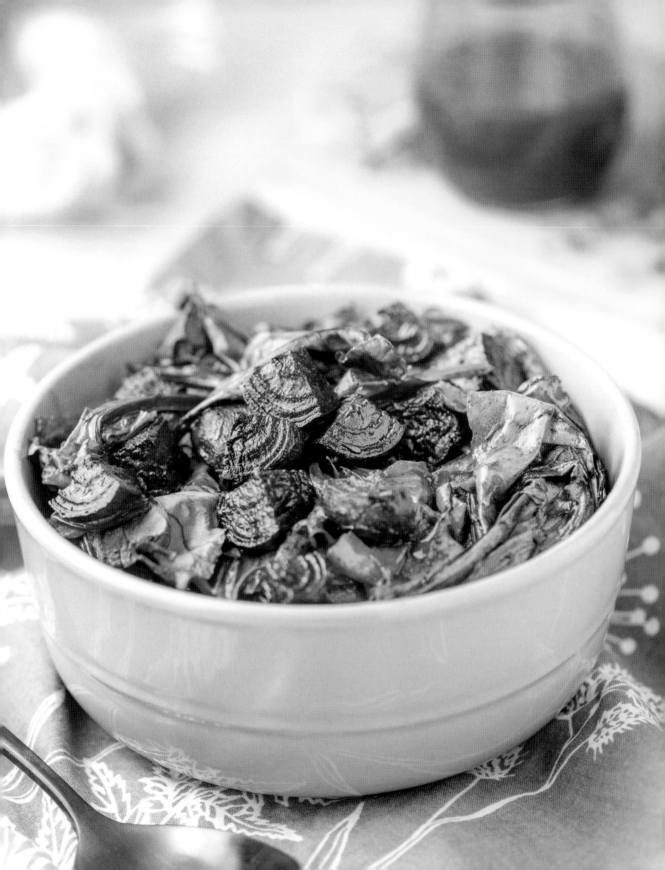

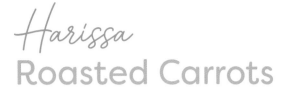
Roasted Carrots

YIELD: 6 servings

PREP TIME: 10 minutes

COOK TIME: 30 minutes

I love spicy foods, so harissa makes a frequent appearance in my meals. It is a Tunisian hot chile paste (also sold in powder form) that is common in North African cuisine. Because the blends aren't constant, the spiciness varies across brands— something to keep in mind if it's your first time using this peppery paste!

While carrots are typically not thought of as a keto vegetable, I like to work them into my macros every chance I can, not only because of their high levels of carotenoids but also because I think they're delicious. Their natural sweetness helps to tame the heat of harissa; adding a touch of sugar-free maple syrup or honey can cut the intensity even more. If you're making this dish for a higher-carb day, go for the real stuff!

¼ cup (60ml) extra-virgin olive oil

1 tablespoon harissa paste or powder

¼ teaspoon garlic powder

¼ teaspoon salt

12 ounces (340g) carrots, sliced on the diagonal

1 tablespoon lemon juice

2 tablespoons chopped shelled raw pistachios, for garnish

2 tablespoons chopped fresh parsley, for garnish

- Preheat the oven to 375°F (190°C).

- In a large bowl, whisk together the oil, harissa, garlic powder, and salt. Toss the carrots in the oil mixture until completely coated. Transfer the carrots to a roasting pan with a lid or a Dutch oven. Cover and roast for 15 minutes.

- Stir the carrots to redistribute the oil and seasoning. Return the pan to the oven and roast uncovered for another 15 minutes, until the carrots are easily pierced with a knife.

- Toss the carrots with the lemon juice and transfer to a serving dish. Sprinkle with the pistachios and parsley to serve.

TO STORE: Refrigerate in an airtight container for up to 3 days.

TO REHEAT: Warm in a small frying pan over low heat for about 5 minutes, until the desired temperature is reached.

MAKE IT MEDIUM-CARB: Whisk in 2 tablespoons maple syrup or honey with the oil, harissa, garlic powder, and salt.

NUTRITION:
138 calories | **11.4g** fat | **1.8g** protein | **8.4g** total carbs | **5.4g** net carbs

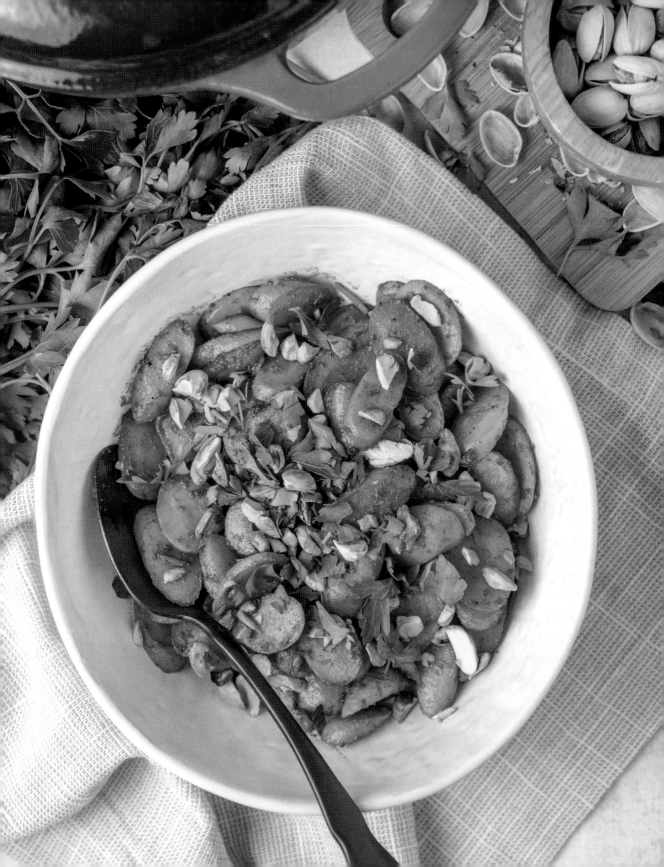

Roasted Lemon-Pepper Asparagus

YIELD: 3 servings

PREP TIME: 5 minutes

COOK TIME: 15 minutes

Nothing says spring to me more than asparagus. While you can technically find asparagus in grocery stores throughout the year, I think it's best when it's in season. Asparagus is very low in carbohydrates, making it a perfect option for keto meals. It's also pretty delicious without needing too much gussying up; a simple lemon-pepper seasoning really makes it shine.

1 bunch medium-thick asparagus (about 1 pound/ 454g)

2 tablespoons extra-virgin olive oil

1 tablespoon grated lemon zest

½ teaspoon ground black pepper

¼ teaspoon salt

- Preheat the oven to 375°F (190°C) and line a rimmed baking sheet with parchment paper.

- Prep the asparagus by removing the woody part of the stems, then place on the baking sheet so the spears are lined up in the same direction.

- In a small bowl, whisk together the oil, zest, pepper, and salt and pour the mixture over the asparagus. Roll the asparagus around on the baking sheet so that the spears are evenly coated in the oil. Bake for 12 to 15 minutes, until the asparagus is tender and can easily be pierced with a knife.

TO STORE: Refrigerate in an airtight container for up to 3 days.

TO REHEAT: Warm in a small frying pan over low heat for about 5 minutes, until the desired temperature is reached.

NUTRITION:
103 calories | **9.1g** fat | **2.5g** protein | **4.6g** total carbs | **2.1g** net carbs

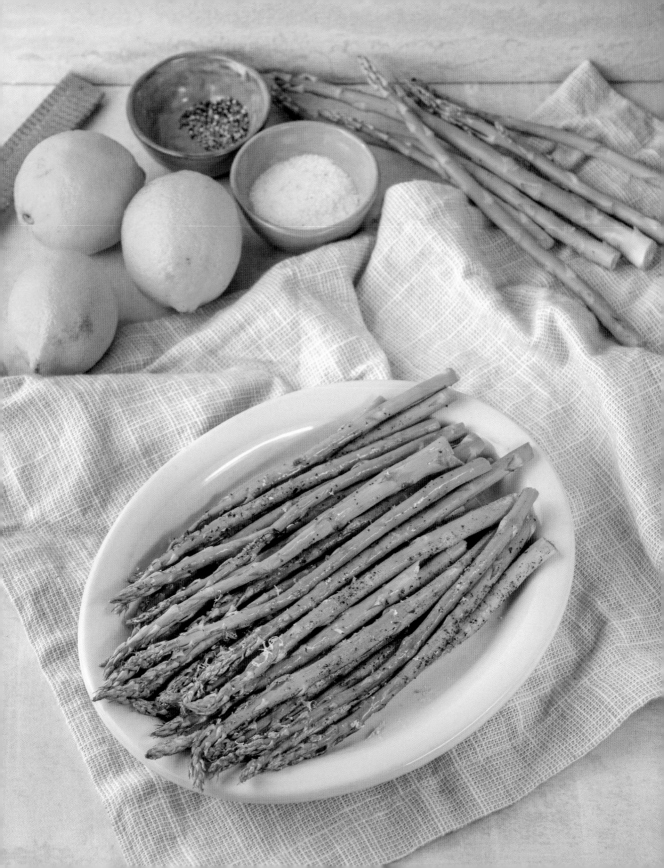

Chimichurri Roasted Celeriac

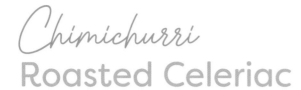

YIELD: 3 servings

PREP TIME: 10 minutes
(not including time to make
chimichurri)

COOK TIME: 40 minutes

If you're not familiar with chimichurri, you're missing out. The pestolike Argentine sauce is absolutely delicious and makes everything it touches even more delicious—especially celeriac. In my quest to find low-carb potato replacements, I've become quite attached to celeriac, also known as celery root. The bulb does taste like celery, but I enjoy that. And while it is a little higher in carbs than most keto-friendly vegetables, it's nice to have variety.

If you can't find celeriac, don't like celery, or want a lower-carb option, I highly recommend using cauliflower or broccoli florets instead (see the variations below). They're just as delicious and have even more favorable keto macros.

1 small celery root (about 8 ounces/225g), peeled and cubed

1 tablespoon extra-virgin olive oil

1 teaspoon crushed or minced garlic

1 teaspoon chili powder

¼ teaspoon salt

2 tablespoons Chimichurri (page 242)

Red pepper flakes, for garnish

- Preheat the oven to 375°F (190°C) and line a rimmed baking sheet with parchment paper or a silicone baking mat.

- In a medium bowl, toss the cubed celery root with the oil, garlic, chili powder, and salt until completely coated. Spread the celery root on the lined baking sheet and roast for 35 to 40 minutes, until soft on the inside.

- Remove from the oven, return to the bowl, and toss with the chimichurri. Garnish with red pepper flakes and serve.

TO STORE: Refrigerate in an airtight container for up to 3 days.

TO REHEAT: Warm in a preheated 300°F (150°C) oven for about 5 minutes, until warmed through.

VARIATIONS:

Chimichurri Roasted Cauliflower. Use 8 ounces (225g) cauliflower florets in place of the celeriac and bake for 30 to 35 minutes, until the florets are tender.

Chimichurri Roasted Broccoli. Use 8 ounces (225g) broccoli florets in place of the celeriac and bake for 20 to 25 minutes, until the florets are tender.

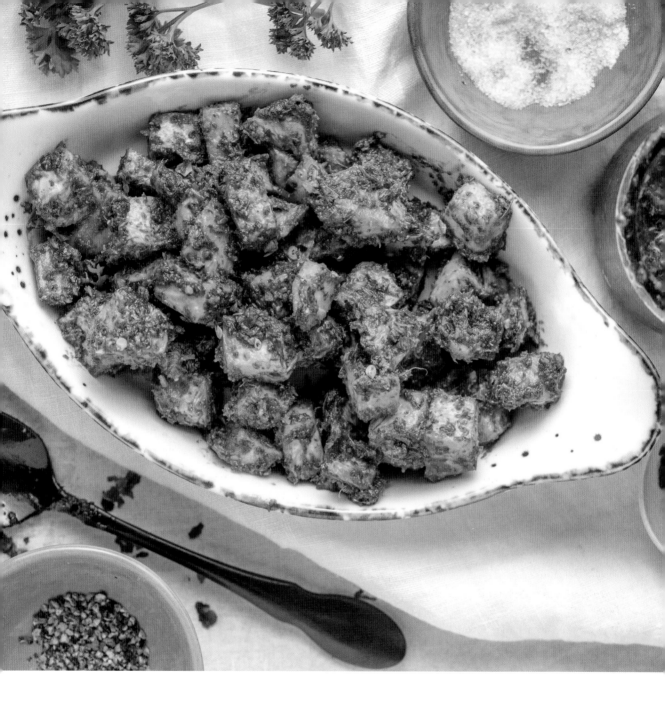

NUTRITION:
111 calories | **8.6g** fat | **1.4g** protein | **7.9g** total carbs | **4.7g** net carbs

NUTRITION (CHIMICHURRI ROASTED CAULIFLOWER):
98 calories | **8.6g** fat | **1.7g** protein | **4.7g** total carbs | **2.7g** net carbs

NUTRITION (CHIMICHURRI ROASTED BROCCOLI):
101 calories | **8.5g** fat | **2.6g** protein | **5g** total carbs | **2.2g** net carbs

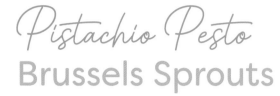
Pistachio Pesto Brussels Sprouts

YIELD: 6 servings

PREP TIME: 5 minutes (not including time to make pesto)

COOK TIME: 20 minutes

I find it a little odd that many people claim to dislike Brussels sprouts. They are so darn delicious, especially with a healthy dose of fat and salt! I love shaved Brussels sprouts for two reasons:

1) I can buy them this way when I'm low on time.

2) There are more bits that get crispy in the oven.

Win-win!

12 ounces (340g) shaved Brussels sprouts

½ cup (120ml) plus 2 tablespoons Pistachio Parsley Pesto (page 246), divided

2 tablespoons coarsely chopped shelled raw pistachios

Red pepper flakes, for garnish (optional)

- Preheat the oven to 375°F (190°C) and line a rimmed baking sheet with parchment paper.

- In a large bowl, toss the Brussels sprouts with ½ cup (120ml) of the pesto until completely coated. Spread in a single layer on the lined baking sheet.

- Bake for 20 minutes, or until the sprouts start to brown at the edges and are tender enough to easily be pierced with a knife.

- Transfer the Brussels sprouts to a serving dish and top with the remaining 2 tablespoons of pesto and the chopped pistachios. Garnish with red pepper flakes, if desired.

TO STORE: Refrigerate in an airtight container for up to 3 days.

TO REHEAT: Warm in a small frying pan over low heat for about 5 minutes, until the desired temperature is reached.

NUTRITION:
181 calories | 15.6g fat | 4.3g protein | 8.5g total carbs | 5g net carbs

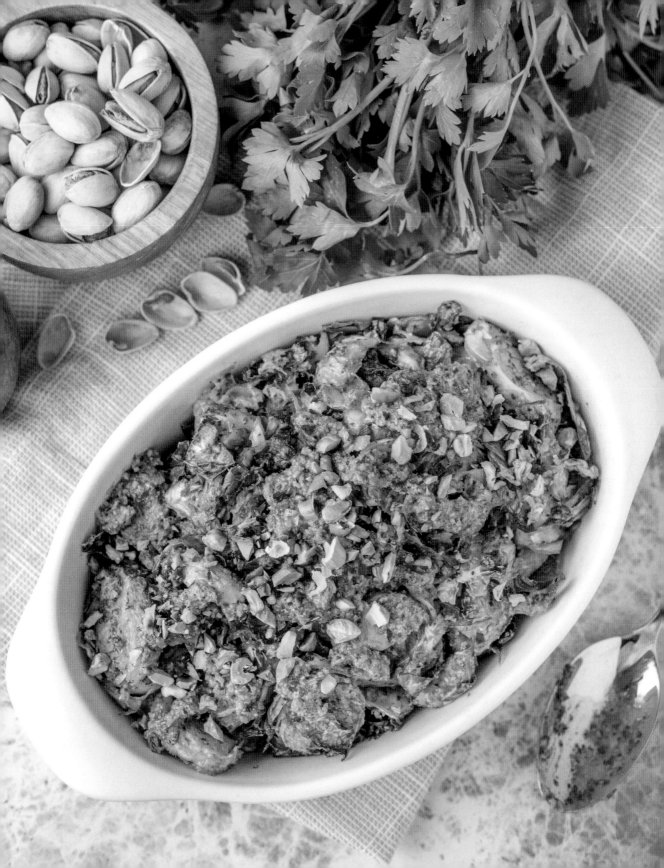

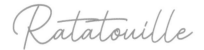

YIELD: 6 servings

PREP TIME: 10 minutes

COOK TIME: 50 minutes

I discovered my love for ratatouille just last year, when I decided to make a French-inspired, travel-themed stay-at-home date night with my husband. I usually make recipes with fairly simple steps and was a little intimidated at how fancy ratatouille looks, with its layers of sliced vegetables. Well, it turns out that it really doesn't take that long. Furthermore, there is no need to arrange them in a pretty spiral as shown. I often just place the slices in rows in a square baking dish.

Ratatouille is a delicious, vegetable-based comfort food that is a terrific side to many proteins. My favorite pairing is the lemon-pepper variation of Basic Baked Tofu (page 170). I also love piling ratatouille on top of a toasted slice of keto-friendly bread for a cozy snack.

4 tablespoons (60ml) extra-virgin olive oil, divided

½ small bell pepper, any color (about 1¼ ounces/35g), cored, seeded, and diced

½ small onion (about 1¼ ounces/35g), diced

¾ teaspoon salt, divided

1 cup (240ml) low-sugar tomato sauce

2 large Roma tomatoes (about 3½ ounces/100g each), thinly sliced

1 medium zucchini (about 7 ounces/200g), thinly sliced

½ small eggplant (about 8 ounces/225g), thinly sliced

1 tablespoon herbes de Provence

¼ teaspoon ground black pepper

- Preheat the oven to 375°F (190°C).

- Heat 1 tablespoon of the oil in a small frying pan over medium-low heat. Add the bell pepper, onion, and half of the salt. Cook, stirring occasionally, until soft, about 5 minutes. Remove from the heat and stir in the tomato sauce.

- Spread the tomato sauce mixture over the bottom of a 1½-quart (1.5-liter) baking dish. Arrange the tomatoes, zucchini, and eggplant slices across the bottom of the pan. (For a pretty presentation, stand the slices on their sides, nestling them in closely; this is particularly pretty in a round baking dish.)

- Whisk the remaining 3 tablespoons of oil with the herbes de Provence, black pepper, and remaining salt and pour the mixture over the vegetables.

- Cover the dish and bake for 30 minutes. Uncover and bake for an additional 15 minutes, until the vegetables are tender and can easily be pierced with a knife.

TO STORE: Refrigerate in an airtight container for up to 4 days.

TO REHEAT: Warm in a preheated 300°F (150°C) oven for about 5 minutes, until the desired temperature is reached.

NUTRITION:
134 calories | 11.9g fat | 1.4g protein | 6.7g total carbs | 4.7g net carbs

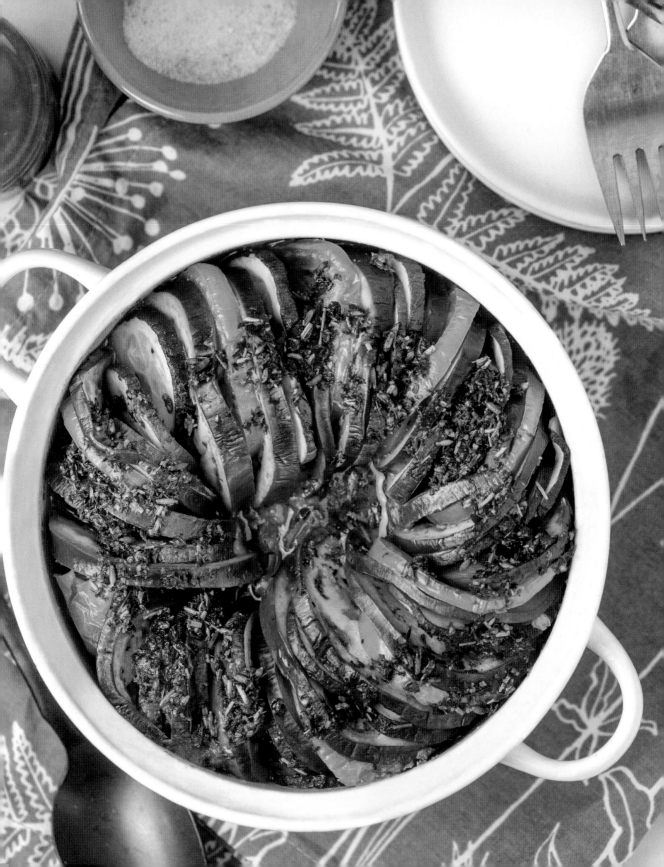

Broccoli Tots

YIELD: 4 servings

PREP TIME: 10 minutes

COOK TIME: 35 minutes

Growing up, I got super excited anytime the school cafeteria served tater tots. As an adult, I still have that same enthusiasm for anything in "tot" form. While cauliflower is an obvious choice for keto tater tots, I think broccoli is a much more flavorful option. If you really dislike broccoli, though, go ahead and use cauliflower.

I usually whip up some Yogurt Dill Sauce (page 240) to dip these in, but store-bought vegan ranch dressing is also a delicious option.

3 cups (210g) broccoli florets

¼ cup (64g) tahini

¼ cup (16g) nutritional yeast

¼ teaspoon salt

2 tablespoons water (if needed)

1 tablespoon psyllium husks

- Preheat the oven to 375°F (190°C) and line a rimmed baking sheet with parchment paper.

- In a food processor, blend the broccoli, tahini, nutritional yeast, and salt until mostly smooth. Add the water if the ingredients aren't blending smoothly. Remove the blade and stir in the psyllium husks. Let the mixture sit for about 5 minutes to thicken and to allow the psyllium to set up.

- Using a tablespoon, scoop the mixture into 24 tots and place them on the lined baking sheet, leaving space between them. Bake for 30 to 35 minutes, until the tots are golden and crispy.

TO STORE: Refrigerate in an airtight container for up to 4 days.

TO REHEAT: Warm in a preheated 300°F (150°C) oven for 5 minutes, or until warmed through.

NUTRITION:
79 calories | 5.1g fat | 4.7g protein | 5.7g total carbs | 2.9g net carbs

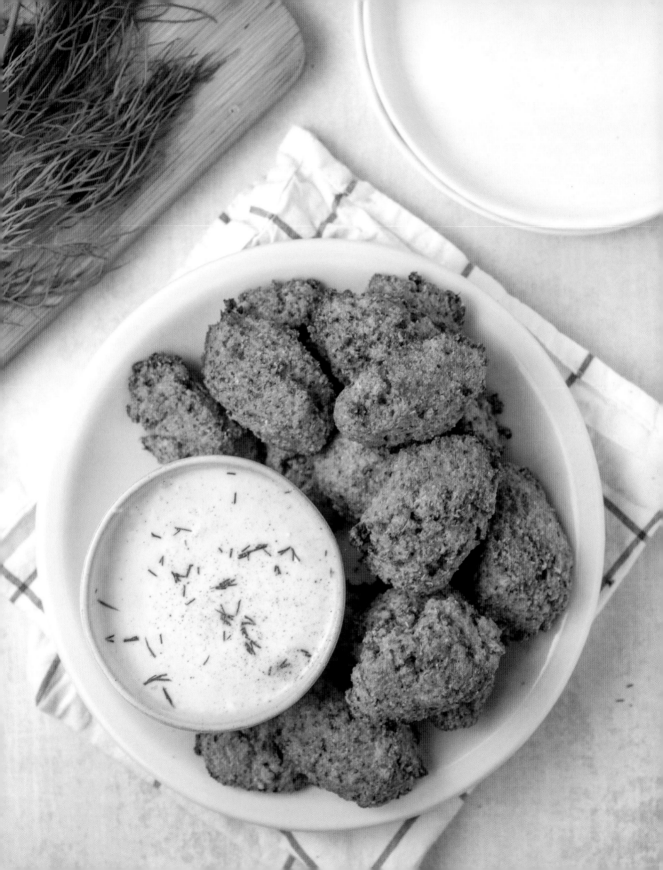

Ras el Hanout
Mashed Butternut Squash

YIELD: 4 servings

PREP TIME: 10 minutes

COOK TIME: 6 or 15 minutes, depending on method

I wasn't the biggest fan of mashed vegetables until I started mashing butternut squash. The squash is so sweet and flavorful on its own that I would happily eat a whole bowl. This keto-friendly version includes cauliflower, but don't worry if it's not your favorite vegetable—you can't even taste it!

Ras el hanout is a delicious and warming North African spice blend. Like many other spice blends, the exact composition varies, and each spice purveyor may have its own recipe. If you can't track down this delicious blend, you can substitute an equal amount of garam masala or make the pumpkin spice variation, opposite.

1 cup (200g) cubed butternut squash

2 cups (200g) cauliflower florets

⅔ cup or 1 cup (160ml or 240ml) vegetable broth, depending on method

2 tablespoons extra-virgin olive oil

2 teaspoons ras el hanout

¼ teaspoon salt

SUGGESTED GARNISHES

Fresh cracked black pepper

Additional ras el hanout

Sliced almonds (omit for nut-free)

- **To make on the stovetop:** In a Dutch oven or other heavy lidded pot over medium heat, bring the squash, cauliflower, and ⅔ cup broth to a simmer. Continue to simmer, covered, for 10 minutes, until the vegetables are soft enough to easily be pierced with a knife. Remove from the heat and drain off any excess liquid.

- **To make in a pressure cooker:** Combine the squash, cauliflower, and 1 cup broth in a pressure cooker. Cook on high pressure for 6 minutes, then let the pressure release naturally. Drain the vegetables of any remaining broth.

- Transfer the squash and cauliflower to a blender or food processor. Add the oil, ras el hanout, and salt and blend until smooth. Transfer the mash to a serving bowl and garnish as desired.

TO STORE: Refrigerate in an airtight container for up to 3 days, or freeze for up to a month.

TO REHEAT: Warm in a covered saucepan over medium heat until the desired temperature is reached.

MAKE IT MEDIUM-CARB: Replace the cauliflower with an additional 2 cups (400g) of butternut squash.

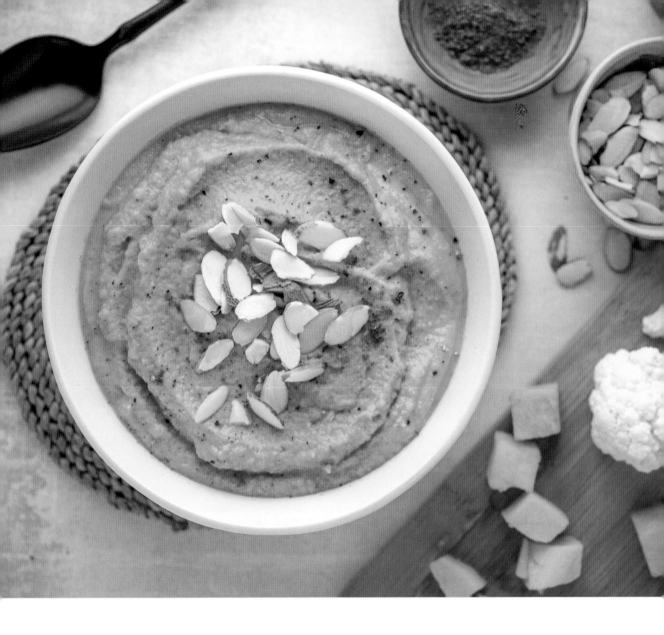

VARIATION: Pumpkin Spice Mashed Butternut Squash. Replace the olive oil with ¼ cup (64g) unsweetened, unsalted almond butter and the ras el hanout with an equal amount of pumpkin pie spice.

NUTRITION:
97 calories | **7g** fat | **1.5g** protein | **8.5g** total carbs | **5.6g** net carbs

NUTRITION (PUMPKIN SPICE MASHED BUTTERNUT SQUASH):
134 calories | **8.9g** fat | **4.8g** protein | **11.4g** total carbs | **6.9g** net carbs

Tofu Fries

YIELD: 5 servings

PREP TIME: 10 minutes

COOK TIME: 40 minutes

I had been vegan for many years before discovering the joy that is a plateful of tofu fries: it was love at first sight. Tofu fries are super easy to make, low in carbs, and high in protein. While they crisp up nicely in the oven, using an air fryer gets them crispy in half the time with no flipping halfway through. Either way, they are beyond delicious.

You can dip these fries in just about any low-carb sauce your heart desires. I like to whip up some Green Goddess Dressing (page 241) or Chimichurri (page 242) or pull out a dairy-free ranch dressing. Sugar-free BBQ sauce is another great option.

Using previously frozen and thawed tofu (see page 172) gives the fries some extra texture, but it's not a necessity.

1 (14-ounce/397-g) block extra-firm tofu

2 tablespoons extra-virgin olive oil

½ teaspoon salt

¼ teaspoon garlic powder

Dipping sauce of choice, for serving

TO STORE: Refrigerate in an airtight container for up to 4 days.

TO REHEAT: Warm in a preheated 300°F (150°C) oven for about 5 minutes, until warmed through.

TO MAKE IN AN AIR FRYER: Place the coated strips in the air fryer tray and air-fry at 375°F (190°C) for 18 to 20 minutes, until completely crispy.

- Preheat the oven to 375°F (190°C) and line a rimmed baking sheet with parchment paper.

- Drain the tofu and press out any excess liquid. Pat the outside of the tofu with a clean kitchen towel or paper towels to remove excess moisture. Cut the tofu into ½-inch (1.25-cm) slices, then lay them flat and cut each slice into ½-inch (1.25-cm) strips.

- Place the strips on the lined baking sheet, brush with half of the oil, and sprinkle with half of the salt and garlic powder. Flip them over and repeat this process on the other side.

- Bake for 20 minutes. Turn the strips over and bake for another 20 minutes, or until they are crispy. Let cool slightly and enjoy with a dipping sauce.

VARIATIONS:

BBQ Tofu Fries. Whisk 2 tablespoons sugar-free BBQ sauce in with the olive oil.

Buffalo Tofu Fries. Replace the olive oil with a nondairy butter substitute and add 1 tablespoon hot sauce.

Chili Tofu Fries. Whisk 1 teaspoon chili paste or Sriracha sauce into the oil.

NUTRITION:
124 calories | **9.2g** fat | **8.5g** protein | **3g** total carbs | **2g** net carbs

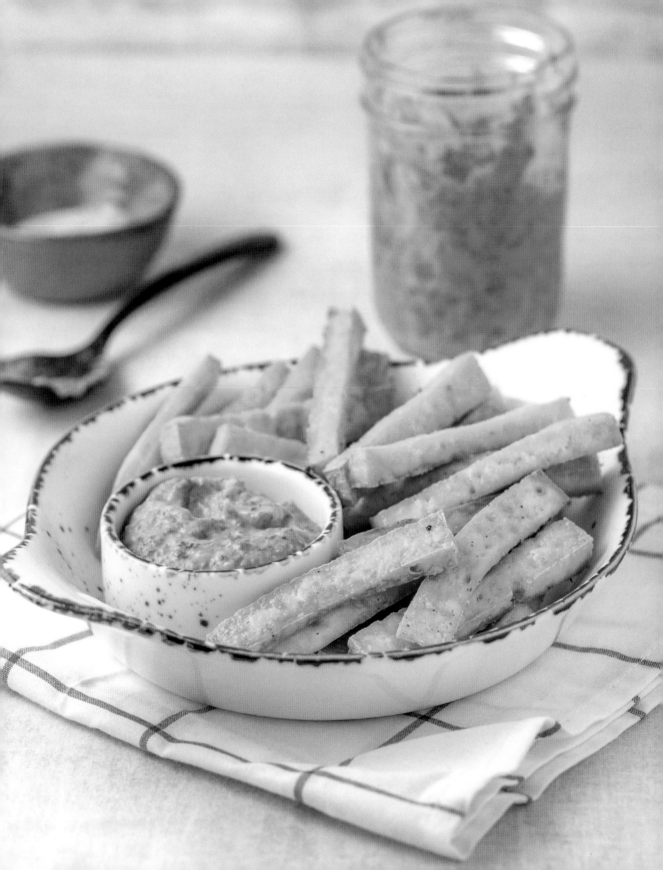

Lupin
Spinach Fritters

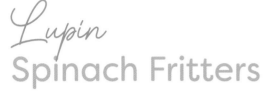

YIELD: 6 fritters (2 per serving)

PREP TIME: 10 minutes

COOK TIME: 12 minutes

I had a hard time figuring out where in the book to place these fritters. While technically they fall in the "small bites" category, they pack loads of protein, and I often eat them as the main part of my meal with some sides. I also sometimes make mini versions (yielding around 24 mini fritters).

While you can use fresh spinach and blanch and drain it, I find that frozen spinach works better for this recipe. Plus, it's a lot less work to go with frozen, prechopped greens. As you may have guessed, you also don't have to limit your greens to spinach. Kale, collard greens, chard, and pretty much any other similar green will work just as well!

6 ounces (170g) frozen chopped spinach, thawed

½ cup (120ml) unsweetened coconut yogurt

½ cup (60g) lupin flour

3 tablespoons extra-virgin olive oil, divided

1 tablespoon prepared yellow mustard

1 tablespoon chopped fresh dill

1 tablespoon psyllium husks

½ teaspoon salt

¼ teaspoon granulated garlic

- In a medium bowl, stir together the spinach, yogurt, lupin flour, 2 tablespoons of the oil, the mustard, dill, psyllium husks, salt, and granulated garlic until a stiff batter forms.

- Heat the remaining 1 tablespoon of oil in a large nonstick frying pan over medium heat, using a brush to distribute the oil.

- Scoop up the batter ¼ cup (60ml) at a time and place in the heated pan. Cook until the undersides of the patties are golden brown, about 7 minutes. Brush the pan with additional oil if needed, flip each patty, flatten with a spatula, and continue cooking for another 5 minutes, until both sides are golden.

TO STORE: Refrigerate in an airtight container for up to 4 days.

TO REHEAT: Warm in a small frying pan over low heat for about 5 minutes, until warmed through.

NUTRITION:
169 calories | **11.9g** fat | **10g** protein | **13.7g** total carbs | **3.1g** net carbs

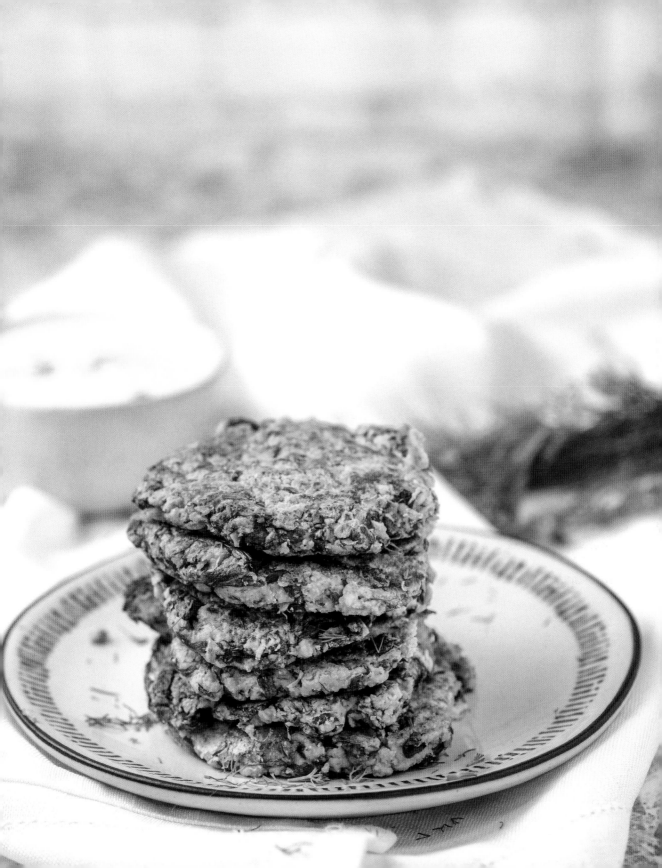

Taco
Fat Bombs

YIELD: 12 fat bombs (1 per serving)

PREP TIME: 5 minutes, plus 30 minutes to chill

I'm a big fan of savory fat bombs. Usually, when I want a snack, I want something savory. I also really like to use these as salad toppings. Adding some fat bombs and dressing to lettuce can take it from a boring bowl of leaves to a filling and delicious lunch.

Make sure to check the ingredients on your taco seasoning, as many include sugar or other hidden carbs! The seasoning blend that I use contains salt, and between that and the salsa, I find that I don't need to add more.

1 cup (120g) chopped raw walnuts

¼ cup (40g) hulled hemp seeds

¼ cup (16g) nutritional yeast

2 teaspoons taco seasoning

Grated zest of 1 lime

2 tablespoons salsa

- Line a rimmed baking sheet with parchment paper.

- In a food processor, blend the walnuts, hemp seeds, nutritional yeast, taco seasoning, and lime zest until a coarse meal forms, 30 to 60 seconds. Add the salsa and blend until a somewhat crumbly "dough" forms, 10 to 20 seconds. It should hold together when pinched.

- Using your hands, roll the mixture into twelve balls, about 1 tablespoon each. Place the balls on the lined baking sheet. Chill in the freezer for at least 30 minutes or in the refrigerator for 2 hours before serving.

TO STORE: Refrigerate in an airtight container for up to a week, or freeze for up to a month.

NUTRITION:
90 calories | **8.2g** fat | **3.2g** protein | **2.5g** total carbs | **1.3g** net carbs

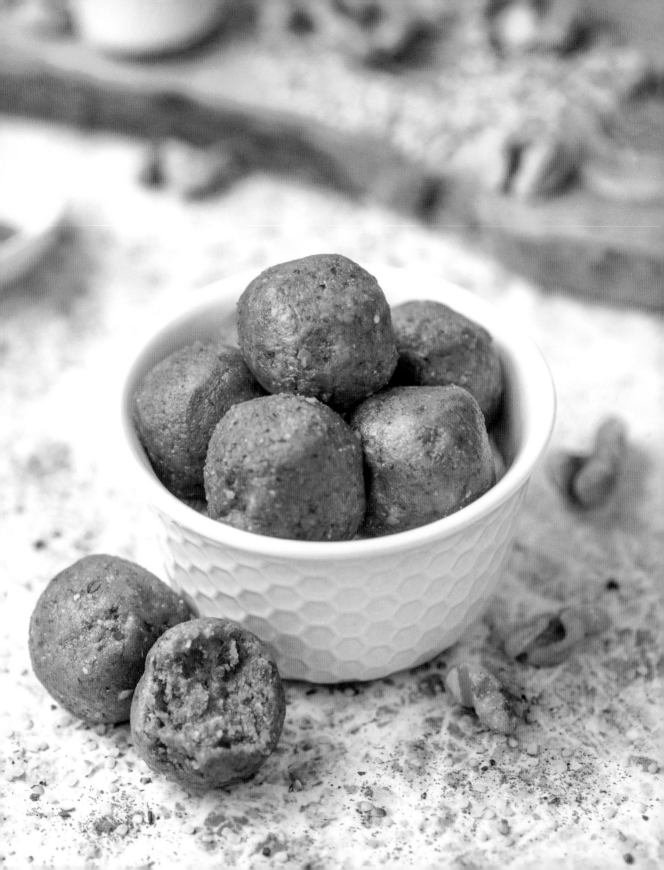

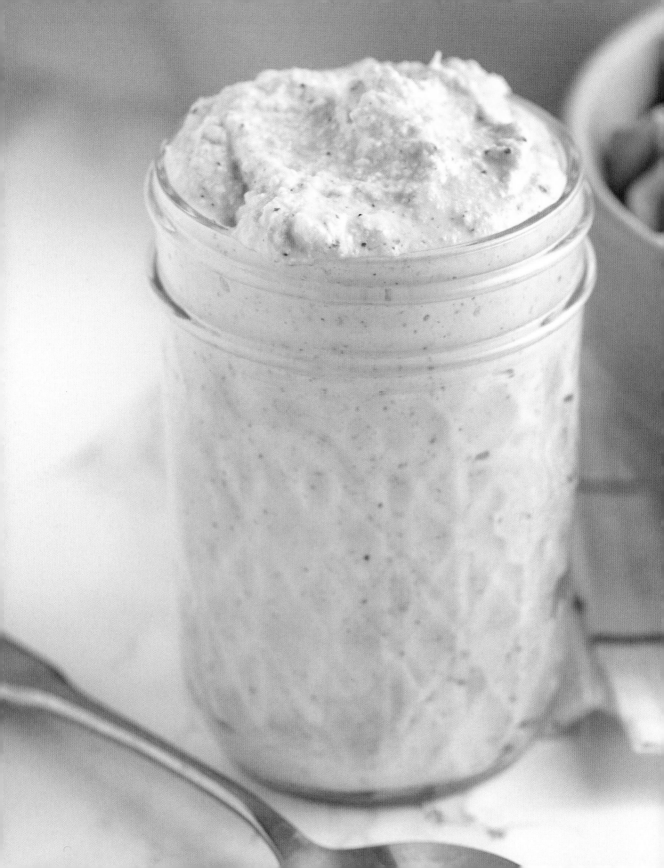

CHAPTER 5:

Sauces & Condiments

Yogurt Dill Sauce

YIELD: 1¼ cups/300ml (¼ cup plus 1 tablespoon/75ml per serving)

PREP TIME: 5 minutes

Dill is my absolute favorite herb. I just adore it and will take any excuse to add it to a meal. I usually use this sauce for dipping falafel (like the Falafel Waffles on page 98), but it's a great dipping sauce for pretty much anything salty and crunchy.

I usually use coconut yogurt, but you can use whatever type of unsweetened yogurt you like best.

1 cup (240ml) unsweetened nondairy yogurt

½ cup (20g) finely chopped fresh dill

2 tablespoons lemon juice

½ teaspoon minced garlic

¼ teaspoon salt

¼ teaspoon ground white pepper

TO STORE: Refrigerate in a tightly sealed jar for up to 5 days.

In a small dish, whisk together all of the ingredients.

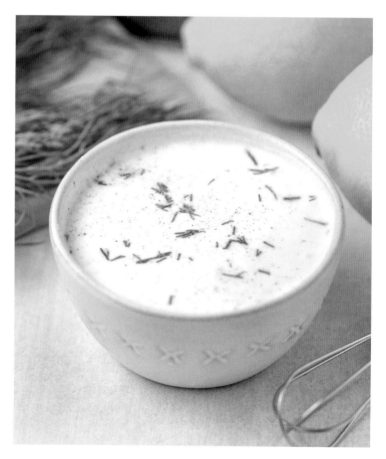

NUTRITION:
31 calories | **1.9g** fat | **0.4g** protein | **3.8g** total carbs | **2.7g** net carbs

Green Goddess
Dressing

YIELD: 2 cups/480ml (¼ cup/60ml per serving)

PREP TIME: 10 minutes

The first time I had green goddess dressing, it was an impulse buy from Trader Joe's. (This is where a lot of my food discoveries begin.) After that, I was hooked. This is my attempt at re-creating that dressing. Aside from using it in Green Goddess Bowls (page 162) and Green Goddess Broccoli Slaw (page 206), I often use it as a dipping sauce for Broccoli Tots (page 228), Tofu Fries (page 232), and Lupin Spinach Fritters (page 234).

One thing I love about this recipe is that it's really versatile. If you are out of chives, you can use scallions. Or, if you don't have any basil left, why not see how it tastes with some mint or dill? You can also play around with the ratios of the herbs with little effect on the macros.

1 medium Hass avocado (about 7½ ounces/212g), halved and pitted

⅔ cup (160ml) water

¼ cup extra-virgin olive oil

Juice of 1 lemon

½ cup (30g) fresh parsley leaves

½ cup (25g) chopped fresh chives

½ cup (20g) fresh basil leaves

1 tablespoon minced garlic

½ teaspoon salt

¼ teaspoon ground black pepper

TO STORE: Refrigerate in a tightly sealed jar for up to 5 days.

Scoop the flesh of the avocado into a blender or food processor. Add the rest of the ingredients and blend until smooth, 1 to 2 minutes.

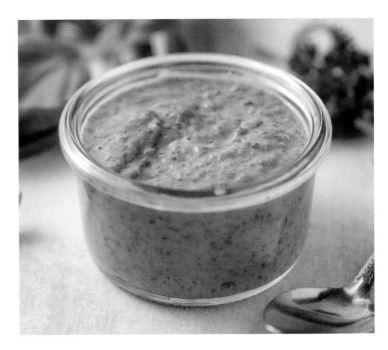

NUTRITION:
94 calories | **9.5g** fat | **0.7g** protein | **2.7g** total carbs | **1.3g** net carbs

Chimichurri

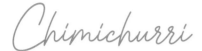

YIELD: ¾ cup/180ml
(2 tablespoons/30ml per serving)

PREP TIME: 5 minutes

Do you ever fall in love with a sauce and then proceed to use it on everything for the next year? That pretty well describes my relationship with chimichurri. I can't stop making it, and I can't stop eating it. You can buy seasoning blends for chimichurri at Latin American food markets and even buy the sauce premade—or you can make your own from scratch! In addition to using this in recipes like Chimichurri Roasted Celeriac (page 222) and Empanada-Inspired Collard Wraps (page 150), I love it as a dip for sliced vegetables and have been known to drizzle it over a bowl of chickpea pasta on a medium-carb day.

This version isn't traditional, but it's how I've been making chimichurri. I've adapted it slightly over the last year or so, and this is the final form. If you're interested in traditional Argentine cuisine, I highly recommend heading to your local library/bookstore/search engine and doing a culinary deep dive.

1 cup (60g) coarsely chopped fresh parsley

4 cloves garlic, peeled

¼ cup plus 1 tablespoon (75ml) extra-virgin olive oil

3 tablespoons red wine vinegar

1 tablespoon dried oregano leaves

½ teaspoon red pepper flakes

½ teaspoon salt

½ teaspoon ground black pepper

TO STORE: Refrigerate in a tightly sealed jar for up to 10 days.

Put all of the ingredients in a blender or food processor and blend until mostly smooth with a few chunks remaining, about 90 seconds.

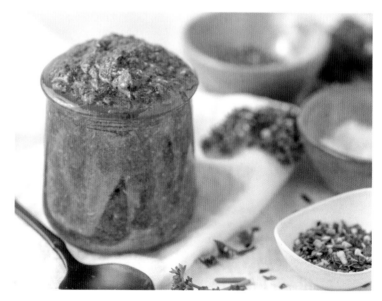

NUTRITION:
107 calories | **11.4g** fat | **0.4g** protein | **1.2g** total carbs | **0.6g** net carbs

Pantry
Peanut Sauce

YIELD: ¾ cup/180ml
(2 tablespoons/30ml per serving)

PREP TIME: 5 minutes

This sauce was born on a trip to Vermont. My husband and I didn't want to go out to dinner, but the ingredients we had on hand in the cabin were pretty limited. We ate this sauce over noodles and broccoli for four nights in a row and then continued to make it at home pretty much every night the next week. It is that good (and we're creatures of habit).

Aside from the lime juice (a later addition), these are ingredients that I always have in my pantry. While this sauce is delicious when used right away, it gets even better when the flavors have time to blend in the refrigerator for a few hours. I most often use it in Peanutty Veggie Noodle Bowls (page 164) and the peanut tempeh variation of the Balsamic-Marinated Skillet Tempeh (page 176). It also makes a great dipping sauce for raw vegetables, especially carrots, celery, and bell peppers.

½ cup (128g) unsweetened creamy peanut butter

¼ cup (60ml) water

Juice of 1 lime

1 tablespoon low-sodium tamari

1 teaspoon chili paste, Sriracha sauce, or other hot sauce

¼ teaspoon granulated garlic, or 1 teaspoon minced garlic

¼ teaspoon ginger powder, or 1 teaspoon grated fresh ginger

TO STORE: Refrigerate in a tightly sealed jar for up to 3 days.

In a small bowl, whisk together all of the ingredients until smooth and creamy.

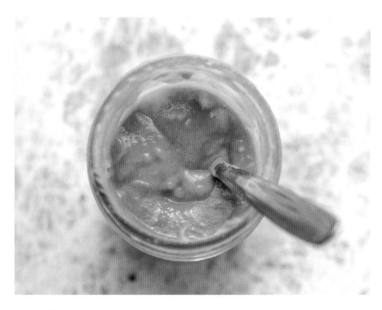

Balsamic
Vinaigrette

YIELD: 1 cup/240ml
(2 tablespoons/30ml per serving)

PREP TIME: 5 minutes, plus
1 hour to chill (optional)

Balsamic vinaigrette is one of my favorite dressings, but it's such a challenge finding a store-bought variety that doesn't contain loads of extra sugar (and low-quality oils, for that matter). So I started making my own. While you can certainly use the vinaigrette immediately after making it, I find that it tastes even better after it's chilled in the refrigerator for an hour.

This is my go-to dressing for easy garden salads as well as my favorite marinade for tempeh (like the Balsamic-Marinated Skillet Tempeh on page 176). I also love tossing some vegetables in the vinaigrette and then roasting them.

¾ **cup (180ml) extra-virgin olive oil**

¼ **cup (60ml) balsamic vinegar**

1 teaspoon Dijon mustard

1 teaspoon crushed garlic

½ **teaspoon dried thyme leaves**

¼ **teaspoon salt**

¼ **teaspoon ground black pepper**

TO STORE: Refrigerate in a tightly sealed jar for up to a week.

In a small bowl, whisk together all of the ingredients. Transfer to a tightly sealed jar or bottle and refrigerate for an hour before serving. Shake the jar before serving.

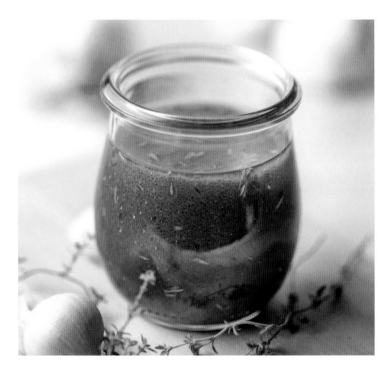

NUTRITION:
187 calories | **20.3g** fat | **0.1g** protein | **1.6g** total carbs | **1.5g** net carbs

Sun-Dried Tomato Dressing

YIELD: ⅔ cup/150ml
(2 tablespoons/30ml per serving)

PREP TIME: 5 minutes

Sun-dried tomatoes, like all dried fruits, are a little higher in carbs than other ingredients, but a little goes a long way. Their flavor is concentrated, so when you blend them into a dressing, it's a relatively low-carb way to enjoy their flavor. I love this as a salad dressing and as a pesto replacement over pasta or on flatbread, like the Veggie Flatbreads on page 140.

I used dry-packed tomatoes. You can use tomatoes that are packed in oil; just be aware that the weight and nutrition information will vary.

¼ cup (15g) sun-dried tomato halves

½ cup (120ml) extra-virgin olive oil

2 tablespoons apple cider vinegar

2 teaspoons chopped garlic

1 teaspoon dried oregano leaves

¼ teaspoon red pepper flakes (optional)

Salt and ground black pepper to taste (see Note)

NOTE: The amount of salt needed will vary depending on the brand of sun-dried tomatoes used.

TO STORE: Refrigerate in a tightly sealed jar for up to 10 days.

Roughly chop the sun-dried tomatoes and place in a blender or food processor with the rest of the ingredients. Blend until smooth, 2 to 3 minutes.

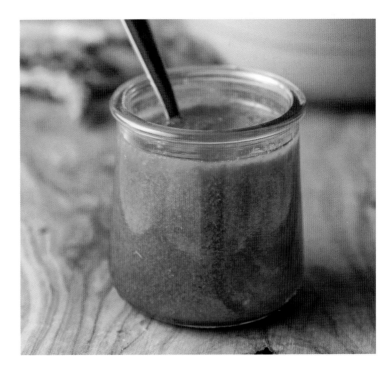

NUTRITION:
201 calories | **21.7g** fat | **0.5g** protein | **2.1g** total carbs | **1.7g** net carbs

Pistachio
Parsley Pesto

YIELD: 1½ cups/350ml
(2 tablespoons/30 ml per serving)

PREP TIME: 5 minutes

2 cups (120g) fresh parsley
leaves

⅔ cup (160ml) extra-virgin
olive oil

½ cup (60g) shelled raw
pistachios

¼ cup (16g) nutritional yeast

2 tablespoons lemon juice

2 cloves garlic, peeled

½ teaspoon salt

TO STORE: Refrigerate in a
tightly sealed jar for up to 10 days.

I am a huge fan of the more widely used basil pesto, but every
once in a while, I like to mix things up with a pistachio parsley
version. I toss it with zucchini noodles, spoon it over baked tofu,
dollop it on veggie burgers, and mix it into roasted vegetables.

Put all of the ingredients in a blender or food processor and blend
until mostly smooth but not completely blended, about 90 seconds.

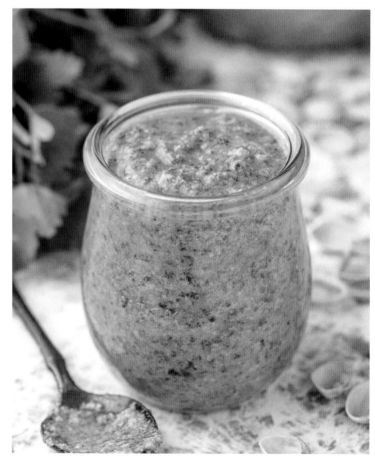

NUTRITION:
172 calories | **17.2g** fat | **2.3g** protein | **3.3g** total carbs | **2g** net carbs

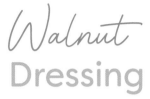

Walnut
Dressing

YIELD: ½ cup plus 2 tablespoons/ 150ml (¼ cup plus 1 tablespoon/ 75ml per serving)

PREP TIME: 10 minutes

My husband is a picky eater, and this dressing is my secret weapon to get him to eat more vegetables. He will eat basically any vegetable when it's topped with this tangy and fresh-tasting dressing. While it's not much to look at, it's delicious!

I mostly use this dressing in the Waldorf Kale Salad on page 132, but it's lovely on any garden salad (or even a simple pile of baby greens).

½ **cup (50g) peeled and cubed jicama**

¼ **cup (30g) chopped raw walnuts**

2 **tablespoons water**

1½ **tablespoons apple cider vinegar**

1½ **tablespoons Dijon mustard**

⅛ **teaspoon salt**

Put all of the ingredients in a blender or food processor and blend until smooth, 30 to 60 seconds. The dressing will be quite thick and spoonable but not pourable.

TO STORE: Refrigerate in a tightly sealed jar for up to 3 days.

MAKE IT MEDIUM-CARB: Replace the jicama with a peeled and cubed medium apple.

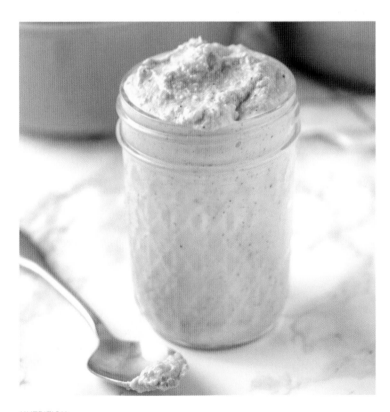

NUTRITION:
122 calories | **10.4g** fat | **3.1g** protein | **5.2g** total carbs | **2.5g** net carbs

Coconut
Fakon Bits

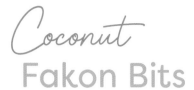

YIELD: ¾ cup/60g
(3 tablespoons/15g per serving)

PREP TIME: 5 minutes

COOK TIME: 25 minutes

One of the weird snacks I used to eat in my teens and twenties was Bac'n Pieces. Yes, you read that correctly. I would eat the crispy, soy-based, fake bacon salad toppers by themselves. I like crunchy things. Anyway, this is my whole food–based version that makes a great salad topper (and snack). If you want to make it soy-free, substitute coconut aminos for the tamari. You can also give it a maple-y flair by adding 1 tablespoon sugar-free maple syrup and baking for an additional 3 to 5 minutes.

¾ cup (60g) unsweetened coconut flakes

1 tablespoon low-sodium tamari

¼ teaspoon smoked paprika

2 tablespoons water

TO STORE: Store in an airtight container for up to a week. I like to toss in a silica packet left over from store-bought kale chips to help keep the coconut as crispy as possible.

- Preheat the oven to 300°F (150°C) and line a rimmed baking sheet with parchment paper.

- Put all of the ingredients in a container, seal tightly, and shake until the coconut has absorbed most of the liquid. I shake for about 15 seconds, let it rest for a minute, and repeat once or twice, about 3 minutes total.

- Spread the coconut in a thin layer on the lined baking sheet and bake until it's dry all the way through and golden around the edges, 20 to 25 minutes (the timing will depend on how thin your coconut flakes are).

NUTRITION:
102 calories | **9.7g** fat | **1.5g** protein | **3.9g** total carbs | **1.4g** net carbs

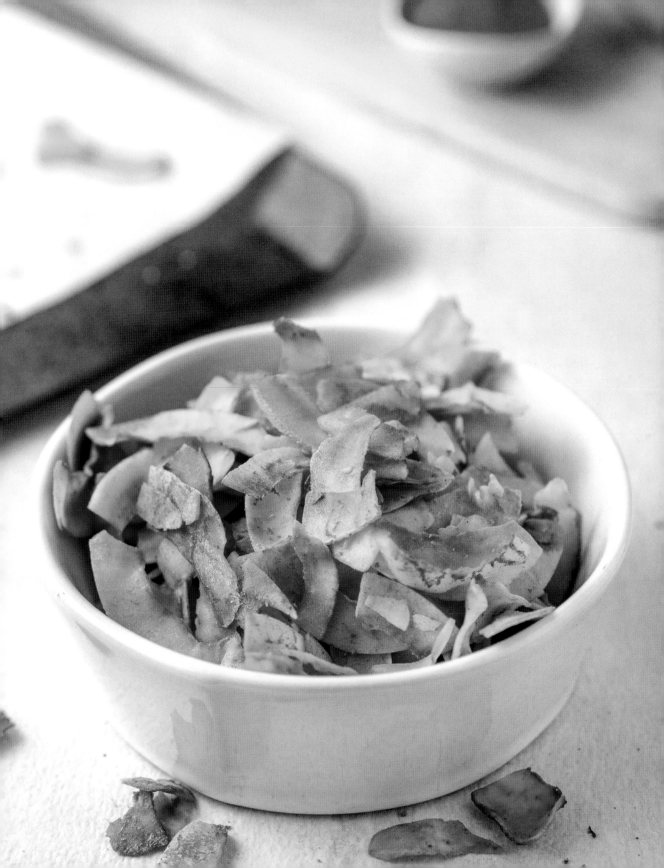

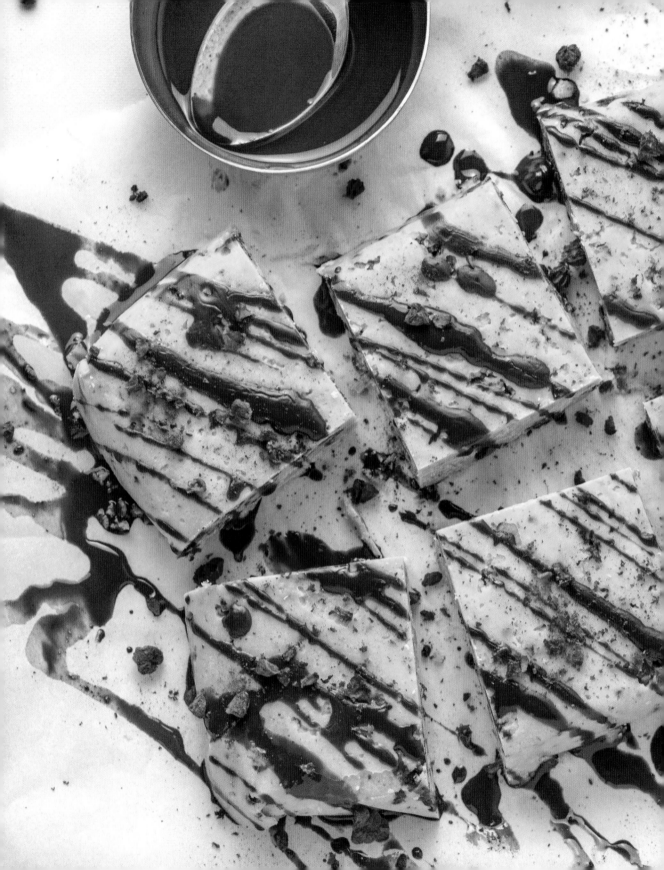

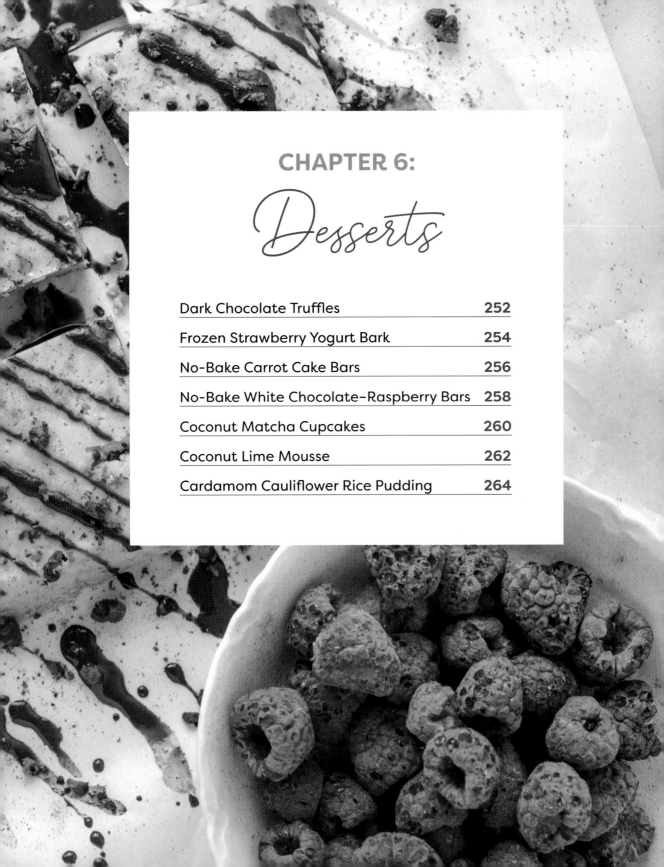

CHAPTER 6:

Desserts

Dark Chocolate Truffles

YIELD: 8 truffles (1 per serving)

PREP TIME: 15 minutes, plus 30 minutes to chill

COOK TIME: 5 minutes

Every year, around the fall and winter holidays, both Trader Joe's and Whole Foods Market sell amazingly rich dark chocolate truffles. My roommates and I would buy boxes of them during those chilly months and eat them as snacks or alongside a cup of hot cocoa—because what goes better with sweet liquid chocolate than sweet solid chocolate? This is my keto-fied version of those sweet treats.

You can use any nut or seed butter you like in place of the almond butter. I often use homemade walnut butter and add a teaspoon of cinnamon when I make these truffles in the fall.

¼ cup (64g) unsweetened creamy almond butter

¼ cup (60g) unsweetened chocolate chips

¼ cup (60ml) allulose syrup or other sugar-free syrup (see Note)

⅛ teaspoon salt

Cocoa powder, for dusting (optional)

- Line an 8-inch (20-cm) square brownie pan with parchment or wax paper.

- In a small bowl set over a saucepan of simmering water (or the top part of a double boiler), melt the almond butter, chocolate, syrup, and salt, stirring constantly, until completely combined.

- Scoop the chocolate mixture into tablespoon-sized dollops, place in the lined pan, and chill in the refrigerator for about 15 minutes, until the truffles have firmed up enough to roll.

- Roll each truffle between your hands to form a ball. If you like, roll each ball in the cocoa powder to coat. Chill for an additional 15 to 20 minutes, until firm.

NOTE: I use allulose for these truffles, but any sugar-free syrupy sweetener should do the trick. You can also use 2 tablespoons of your favorite granulated sweetener stirred into 3 tablespoons nondairy milk.

TO STORE: Store in a tightly sealed container at room temperature for up to 5 days, or refrigerate for up to a week.

NUTRITION:
90 calories | **7.9g** fat | **2.5g** protein | **5.9g** total carbs | **1.2g** net carbs

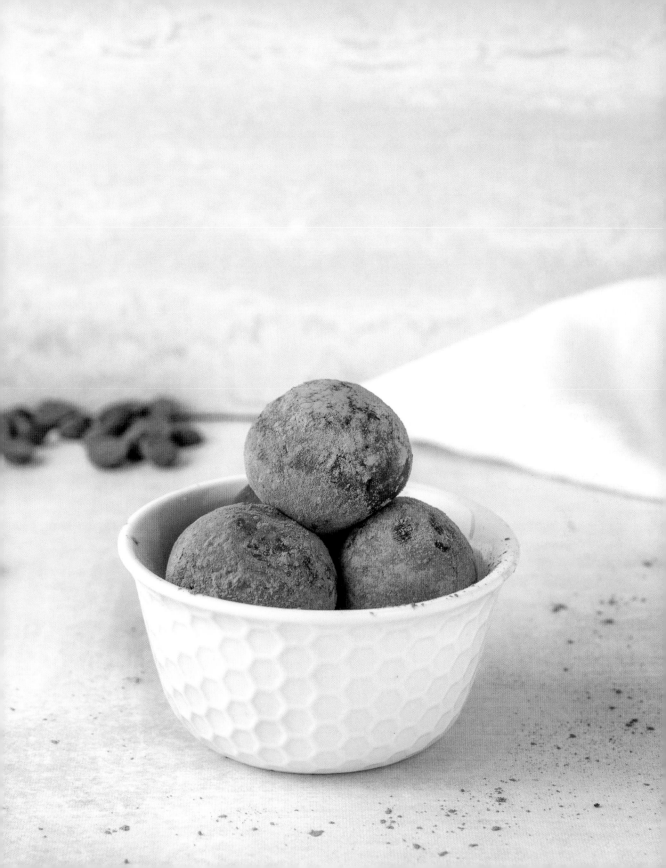

Frozen Strawberry Yogurt Bark

YIELD: 6 servings

PREP TIME: 5 minutes, plus 90 minutes to freeze

I'm not usually a food trends person, but I kept seeing frozen yogurt bark pop up on social media, so I thought I'd give it a try. Since most recipes are pretty high in sugar and low in fat, I had to make some adjustments, but I am super happy with how it turned out—and I'm surprised at how often I make this recipe!

You can use fresh strawberries, but I much prefer freeze-dried berries because they don't freeze into bricks. You can mix in pretty much any nuts and seeds you like instead of the hemp seeds. I also like mixing in cacao nibs, unsweetened chocolate chips, or chopped pistachios or pecans.

1 cup (240ml) unsweetened coconut yogurt

¾ cup (10g) freeze-dried strawberries

¼ cup (60ml) melted coconut oil

¼ cup (40g) hulled hemp seeds

½ teaspoon vanilla extract

⅛ teaspoon liquid stevia

- Line a rimmed baking sheet with parchment paper.

- In a medium bowl, stir together all of the ingredients, breaking up the strawberry bits with the spoon as you mix.

- Spread the mixture evenly on the lined baking sheet; it will be about ½ inch (1.25cm) thick.

- Freeze for about 90 minutes, until the bark is completely frozen. Break into pieces to serve.

TO STORE: Freeze in a covered container for up to a month.

MAKE IT MEDIUM-CARB: Double the amount of freeze-dried strawberries.

NUTRITION:
144 calories | **13.4g** fat | **2.2g** protein | **4g** total carbs | **2.9g** net carbs

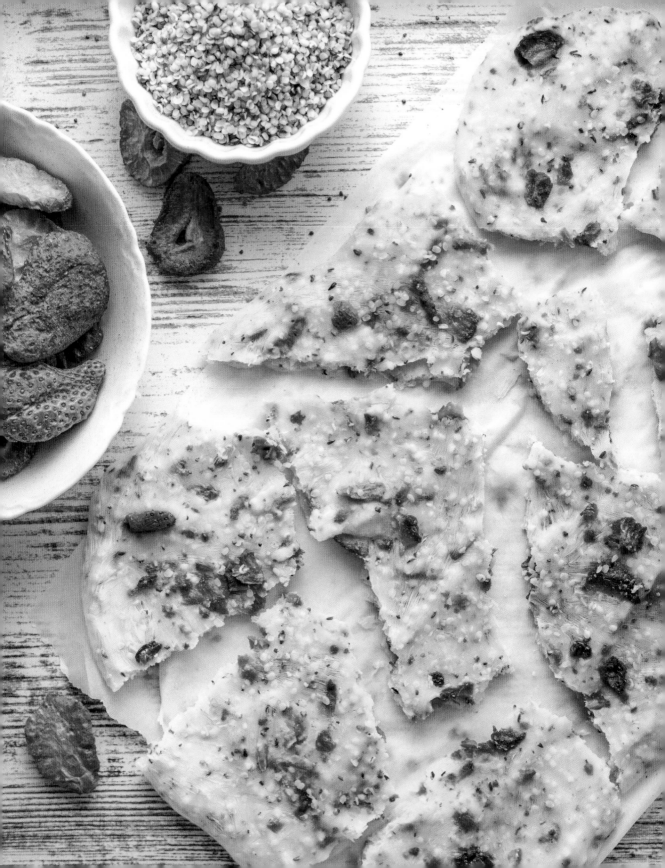

No-Bake Carrot Cake Bars

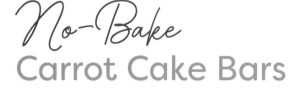

YIELD: 6 large or 9 small bars (1 per serving)

PREP TIME: 5 minutes, plus 4 hours to chill

Although baking is one of my favorite activities, sometimes I want a dessert without having to turn on the oven. I love desserts that seem unhealthy (let's be real—traditional carrot cake is basically a sugar bomb with cream cheese frosting) but are actually nutrient-dense. These bars are just that! They've got the flavors of carrot cake without the excess sugar.

While these bars are delicious after four hours of chilling, I think they taste best if they are refrigerated overnight so all of the flavors meld. We're only human, though, and I know waiting that long for dessert is a big ask!

I usually make the larger size for myself and enjoy one for breakfast with a protein shake, but I often make the smaller size when serving them as a dessert or snack. When I want a little crunch, I chop up additional raw walnuts and lightly press them into the tops of the bars before serving.

1 cup (120g) chopped raw walnuts

1 cup (110g) shredded carrots

½ cup (120g) coconut butter (aka coconut manna)

2 tablespoons lemon juice

2 tablespoons granulated sweetener (see page 69)

1 teaspoon vanilla extract

2 teaspoons ground cinnamon, or grated zest of 1 lemon

Pinch of salt

SPECIAL EQUIPMENT (optional):

6-cavity extra-large silicone ice cube tray (2-inch/5-cm cubes)

- Line an 8-inch (20-cm) square brownie pan with parchment paper. Alternatively, if making large bars, have on hand a silicone ice cube tray with six 2-inch (5-cm) wells.

- Put all of the ingredients in a food processor and process until smooth, about 3 minutes, scraping down the sides as necessary.

- Spread the mixture evenly in the lined brownie pan. Or, if using an ice cube tray, divide the mixture evenly among the wells of the tray. Chill in the refrigerator for at least 4 hours (preferably overnight), until set.

- Slice into 9 small bars or remove the large bars from the ice cube tray to serve.

TO STORE: Refrigerate in an airtight container for up to 5 days, or freeze for up to a month.

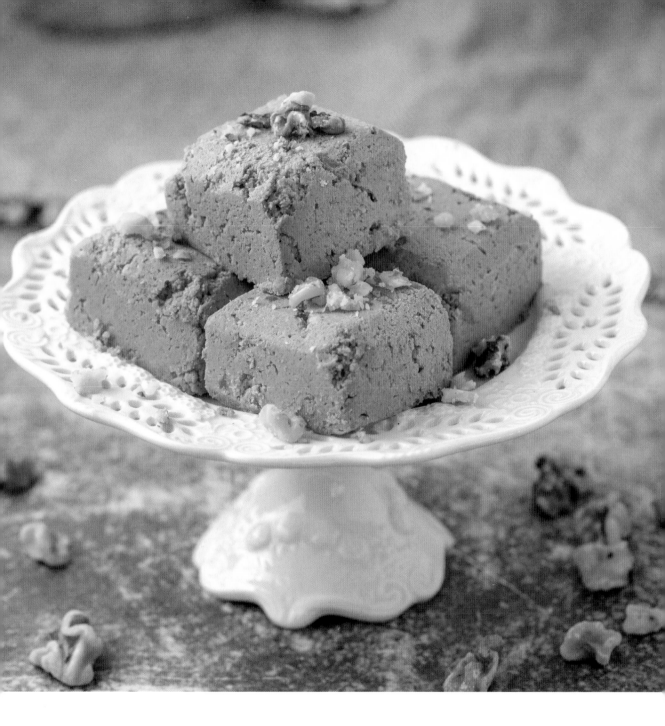

NUTRITION (small bars):
191 calories | **17.3g** fat | **3.1g** protein | **9.3g** total carbs | **2.7g** sugar alcohols | **3.1g** net carbs

NUTRITION (large bars):
286 calories | **26g** fat | **4.7g** protein | **13.9g** total carbs | **4.1g** sugar alcohols | **4.7g** net carbs

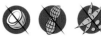

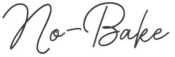
White Chocolate-Raspberry Bars

YIELD: 8 bars (1 per serving)

PREP TIME: 15 minutes, plus 2 hours to chill

COOK TIME: 5 minutes

What I love about no-bake desserts is that they're pretty adaptable to your own tastes because the ratios of ingredients are far less important than in traditional baking. I often make these bars with chocolate protein powder instead of vanilla. I also like to switch out the raspberries for strawberries on occasion. While I use cacao butter for the white chocolate flavor, you could use coconut oil if that's all you have on hand (see Notes).

½ cup (112g) cacao butter

½ cup (128g) nondairy or dairy cream cheese (see Notes), softened

½ cup (60g) vanilla protein powder (see Notes)

½ cup (10g) freeze-dried raspberries

SUGGESTED GARNISHES

Melted sugar-free chocolate, for drizzling

Additional freeze-dried raspberries, crumbled

- Line a 9 by 5-inch (23 by 12.75-cm) loaf pan with parchment paper.

- In a medium bowl set over a saucepan of simmering water (or the top part of a double boiler), melt the cacao butter, then remove from the heat. Add the cream cheese and protein powder and stir until a thick, somewhat crumbly "dough" forms. Stir or knead until the dough is uniform.

- Stir in the raspberries, breaking them up with the spoon so that the pieces are evenly distributed.

- Press the dough into the lined loaf pan. Refrigerate for at least 2 hours, until firm. Slice into 8 bars, garnish as desired, and serve.

NOTES: If you use coconut oil in place of the cacao butter, keep in mind that the bars will soften at a much lower temperature, so they will need to be stored in the freezer to remain firm.

The nondairy cream cheese that I use is a nut-based cream cheese from Miyoko's Creamery. I also like the one from Kite Hill, though any nondairy or dairy cream cheese option will work here.

I use Vega Sport plant-based protein, which is already sweetened. If you are using an unsweetened protein powder, you will want to add a sweetener to taste.

TO STORE: Refrigerate in an airtight container for up to a week, or freeze for up to a month.

NUTRITION:
186 calories | **17.5g** fat | **6.2g** protein | **2.8g** total carbs | **1.6g** net carbs

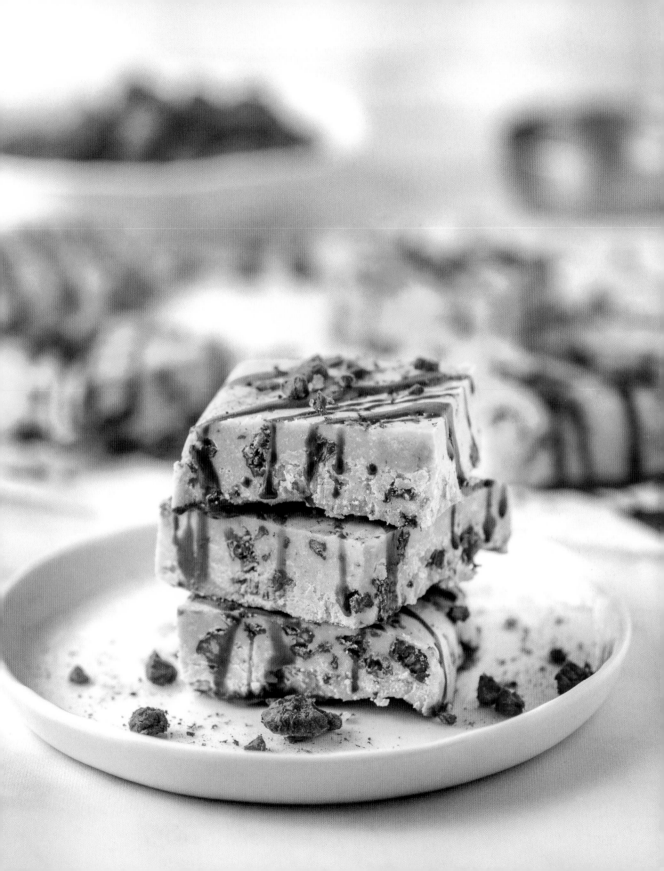

Coconut Matcha Cupcakes

YIELD: 5 cupcakes (1 per serving)

PREP TIME: 15 minutes

COOK TIME: 30 minutes

Coconut and matcha (a ceremonial green tea from Japan) are a lovely combination. These cupcakes taste like a matcha latte to me, just in dessert form. The cake is tender and lightly sweet with the perfect amount of coconut flavor, and the frosting has a delicate matcha taste that balances out the sweetness.

If you can't find matcha powder or don't want to buy an ingredient that you're not sure you'll use again, you can either omit the matcha powder from the frosting or replace it with 1 teaspoon cocoa powder for a lightly chocolatey frosting. I'm not a fan of overly sweet desserts, so I don't add sweetener to the frosting, but you could certainly sweeten it to taste with your favorite sugar-free sweetener.

While it can be hard to wait for the cupcakes to cool before removing them from the pan, they will fall apart if they haven't cooled and set up enough. Have patience!

CUPCAKES

¼ cup (56g) melted coconut butter

½ cup (120ml) lukewarm water or nondairy milk of choice (see Note)

¼ cup (48g) granulated sweetener (see page 69)

1 teaspoon vanilla extract

¼ cup plus 1 tablespoon (35g) coconut flour

2 teaspoons psyllium husks

1 teaspoon baking powder

Pinch of salt

FROSTING

½ cup (120ml) coconut cream

½ teaspoon matcha powder

- **To make the cupcakes:** Preheat the oven to 350°F (177°C). Line five wells of a standard-size muffin pan with paper liners, or have on hand a silicone muffin pan.

- In a small bowl, stir together the coconut butter, water, sweetener, and vanilla until smooth.

- In a separate small bowl, whisk together the coconut flour, psyllium husks, baking powder, and salt until thoroughly combined.

- Fold the dry ingredients into the wet and continue to stir until no clumps remain. Let the batter sit for about 5 minutes so the psyllium starts to gel and the coconut flour absorbs the liquid.

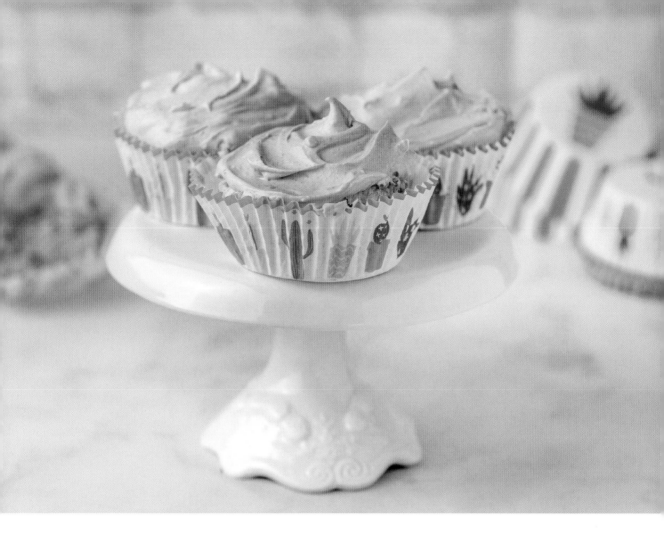

NOTE: The temperature of the water should just be around body temperature so that the coconut butter doesn't harden when mixed. However, it shouldn't be hot enough to prematurely activate the baking powder. While you can use nondairy milk for this recipe, I tend to use water so I can pour it directly from the kettle and don't have to dirty a pan warming milk.

TO STORE: Keep covered at room temperature for up to 2 days (3 days if unfrosted), or refrigerate in an airtight container for up to 5 days.

- Divide the batter evenly among the five muffin wells, filling each one about three-quarters full. Smooth over any peaks with your finger so they don't burn. Bake for 30 minutes, or until the cupcakes are firm to the touch and golden around the edges.

- Let cool in the pan for at least 10 minutes to allow the cupcakes to set up, then carefully move to a cooling rack. Allow to cool completely before removing from the pan and frosting.

- **To make the frosting:** In a small bowl, stir together the coconut cream and matcha powder.

- Once the cupcakes have cooled completely, frost and enjoy.

NUTRITION:
200 calories | **16.7g** fat | **3.1g** protein | **19.4g** total carbs | **9.6g** sugar alcohols | **3.1g** net carbs

Coconut Lime
Mousse

YIELD: 4 servings

PREP TIME: 5 minutes

This is one of those recipes that are so delicious, it's hard to believe they are also so simple. The light and fluffy mousse is perfect on its own, with some garnishes, or as a topping for your favorite dessert! While it is more of a dessert itself, I love mixing in a bunch of hemp seeds (for protein and omega-3s!) and fresh raspberries to have a mousse cup for breakfast.

Any brand of nondairy (or dairy) cream cheese should work here. If you eat dairy, try experimenting with crème fraîche or Neufchâtel in place of the cream cheese to vary the flavor and texture.

1 (8-ounce/225-g) package nondairy cream cheese

1 cup (240ml) coconut cream (or use 1 cup cream from a can of full-fat coconut milk; see page 63)

¼ teaspoon liquid stevia, or ¼ cup (36g) powdered sweetener blend

½ teaspoon vanilla extract (optional)

Juice of 1 lime

SUGGESTED GARNISHES

Hulled hemp seeds

Fresh raspberries

Put the cream cheese, coconut cream, stevia, vanilla (if using), and lime juice in a food processor and blend until smooth, about 1 minute. Portion into four 6-ounce (180-ml) serving cups, garnish as desired, and enjoy.

TO STORE: Cover and refrigerate for up to 5 days.

NUTRITION:
338 calories | **32.1g** fat | **3.3g** protein | **5.6g** total carbs | **5.5g** net carbs

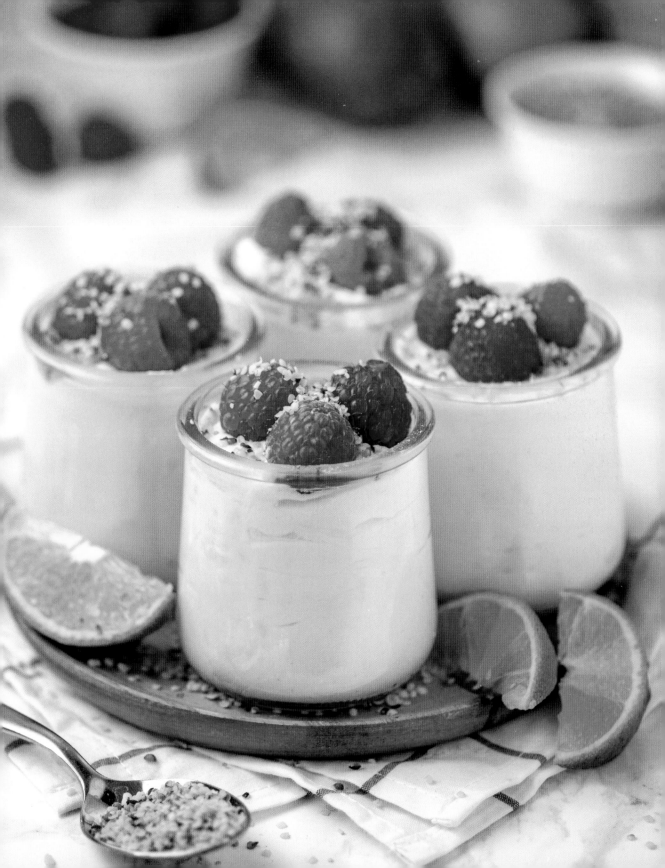

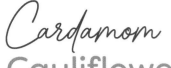
Cardamom
Cauliflower Rice Pudding

YIELD: 3 servings

PREP TIME: 2 minutes

COOK TIME: 20 minutes

I never really gave cardamom a second thought until a Finnish coworker told me that she always adds it to her coffee. So I gave it a try in my coffee and realized I needed a lot more cardamom in my life. This creamy cauliflower rice pudding makes for a perfect dessert or midnight snack, but I've also been known to have a bowl of it for breakfast!

If you aren't a fan of cardamom or don't have any on hand, cinnamon is lovely here as well.

1 (12-ounce/340-g) package frozen riced cauliflower

1 cup (240ml) canned full-fat coconut milk

¼ cup (30g) vanilla protein powder

½ teaspoon ground cardamom

10 drops liquid stevia (optional)

SUGGESTED GARNISHES

Chopped nuts of choice

Sugar-free maple syrup

Sugar-free mock honey (see Note)

Fresh berries

- In a medium saucepan, stir together the riced cauliflower, coconut milk, protein powder, cardamom, and stevia, if using, until combined. Bring to a simmer over medium heat, then cook, stirring frequently, for 15 minutes, until the cauliflower is tender and the pudding has thickened slightly.

- Garnish as desired and serve warm.

NOTE: For a sugar-free honey option, I like Harmless Hunny made by Pyure because it's vegan. But there are many options on the market.

TO STORE: Refrigerate in an airtight container for up to 3 days.

TO REHEAT: Enjoy cold, or warm in a covered saucepan over medium-low heat until the desired temperature is reached.

NUTRITION:
188 calories | **11.7g** fat | **9.1g** protein | **8.5g** total carbs | **5.3g** net carbs

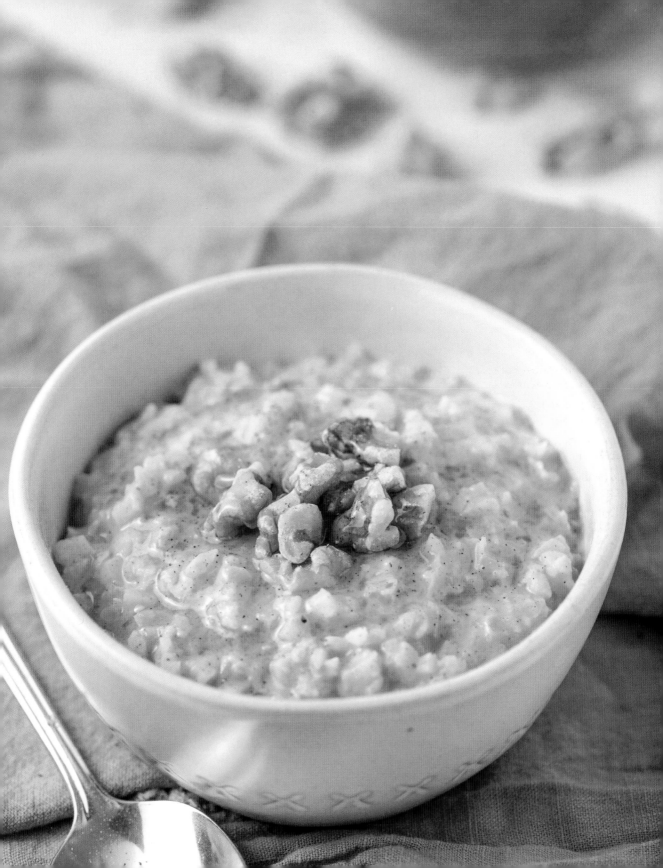

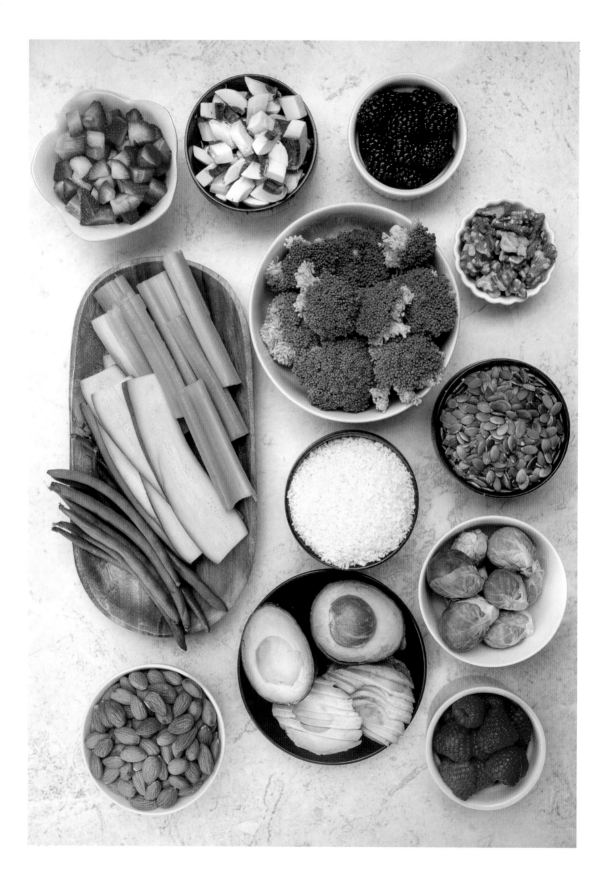

CHAPTER 7:

Meal Plans

- Meal plans are intended only as guidelines and do not need to be followed to the letter. You can (and should) change up the meals and ingredients to meet your macronutrient goals, caloric needs, and taste preferences.

- There are two 4-week plans here. The first plan averages around 1,600 calories and 30 grams of net carbs per day, while the second averages 1,800 calories and 45 grams of net carbs. I chose these targets because they create a caloric deficit for most people, which will facilitate weight loss. If weight loss is not your goal, you can increase the calories by adding more low-carb snacks or loading up your coffee with full-fat coconut milk.

- I have provided a 45-gram net carb plan in addition to the more traditional 30-gram net carb plan for two main reasons. First, I wanted to offer a plan for athletes, people with certain hormonal imbalances, and those of us who menstruate, who tend to feel better eating more carbs. Second, I wanted to show what it might look like to incorporate more carbs in your meals in a moderate way, without heavily processed starches and sugars.

- Weeks 3 and 4 of both plans are entirely soy-free to accommodate those with soy allergies and intolerances. If you cannot consume soy, just start on Week 3 of the plan you wish to follow.

- The protein toppers listed are suggestions based on what I personally would eat with each meal, but you can choose any protein you like. Live your best life!

- When a recipe appears in bold type, it is to be prepared fresh that day. Otherwise, it is meant to be eaten as leftovers.

- When a recipe is followed by a number such as "x2," consume this number of servings. Otherwise, eat one serving as defined in the recipe.

- If you still feel hungry at the end of the day, eat more food! Conversely, if you feel full before eating all of the food on a particular day, don't force it. I include a lot of snacks in my meal plans to give you an easy way to adjust your food intake.

- Although they are not included in the plans, you can drink tea or coffee! Just be sure to prepare it using keto-friendly ingredients; see page 58 for keto-friendly creamer options.

Week 1: ~30g Net Carbs Daily

	Breakfast	Lunch	
Day 1	**Flax Crepes with Avocado & Tomato (page 96) + Tempeh Bacon (page 174)**	**Lupin Spinach Fritters (page 234) + Green Goddess Dressing (page 241)** **Green Goddess Broccoli Slaw (page 206)**	
Day 2	Flax Crepes with Avocado & Tomato + Tempeh Bacon	Peanutty Veggie Noodle Bowl	
Day 3	Flax Crepes with Avocado & Tomato + Tempeh Bacon	Empanada-Inspired Collard Wraps + Chimichurri Green Goddess Broccoli Slaw	
Day 4	**Overnight "N'Oats" (page 104)**	Lupin Spinach Fritters + Green Goddess Dressing Green Goddess Broccoli Slaw	
Day 5	**Pumpkin Spice Breakfast Bars (page 110) (x3)**	Lupin Spinach Fritters + Chimichurri Roasted Lemon-Pepper Asparagus	
Day 6	**PB&J Muffins (page 106) (x2)**	Shepherd's Pie	
Day 7	PB&J Muffins (x2)	Shepherd's Pie	

Dinner	Snacks	Nutrition
Peanutty Veggie Noodle Bowl (page 164)	**Taco Fat Bombs (page 236) (x2)** ½ cup (60g) almonds	**Calories:** 1675 **Fat:** 133.4g **Protein:** 70.6g **Total Carbs:** 82.3g **Net Carbs:** 29.4g
Empanada-Inspired Collard Wraps (page 150) + Chimichurri (page 242) Green Goddess Broccoli Slaw	Taco Fat Bombs (x3)	**Calories:** 1605 **Fat:** 127.3g **Protein:** 73.4g **Total Carbs:** 68.5g **Net Carbs:** 28.2g
Greek Stuffed Pepper (page 148) **Roasted Lemon-Pepper Asparagus (page 220)**	**Dark Chocolate Truffles (page 252) (x4)**	**Calories:** 1611 **Fat:** 123.1g **Protein:** 74.7g **Total Carbs:** 87.7g **Net Carbs:** 30.7g
Greek Stuffed Pepper Roasted Lemon-Pepper Asparagus	Taco Fat Bombs (x2) ½ cup (60g) almonds Dark Chocolate Truffles (x2)	**Calories:** 1618 **Fat:** 128.1g **Protein:** 72.3g **Total Carbs:** 80.3g **Net Carbs:** 29.7g
Shepherd's Pie (page 158)	Taco Fat Bombs (x3)	**Calories:** 1624 **Fat:** 132.2 **Protein:** 77.1g **Total Carbs:** 65.4g **Net Carbs:** 30g
Cabbage Noodle Chow Mein (page 152) + Basic Baked Tofu (page 170)	Pumpkin Spice Breakfast Bars (x3) Taco Fat Bombs (x2)	**Calories:** 1613 **Fat:** 130.8g **Protein:** 73.1g **Total Carbs:** 69g **Net Carbs:** 29.5g
Cabbage Noodle Chow Mein + Basic Baked Tofu	Pumpkin Spice Breakfast Bars (x3) Dark Chocolate Truffles (x2)	**Calories:** 1612 **Fat:** 130.2g **Protein:** 71.7g **Total Carbs:** 75.7g **Net Carbs:** 29.2g

Week 1 Notes

Day 1: Freeze half of the Green Goddess Dressing and Chimichurri and the remaining Pantry Peanut Sauce for Week 2. Save the lime zest from making the Pantry Peanut Sauce for the Taco Fat Bombs.

Day 2: Freeze half of the plant-based ground for Week 3.

Day 3: Freeze half of the Greek Stuffed Peppers for Week 2. Make a double batch of the Dark Chocolate Truffles and freeze half for Week 2.

Day 6: Set aside a PB&J Muffin for Week 2. Freeze half of the Cabbage Noodle Chow Mein and Basic Baked Tofu for Week 2.

Week 1 Ingredients

Produce:

asparagus, 1 bunch (about 1 pound/454g)

basil, 1 small bunch

bell peppers, yellow, orange, or red, 2 large (about 3 inches/7.5cm in diameter) and 1 small (about 2½ ounces/70g)

broccoli slaw, 12-ounce (340-g) package

cabbage, 4 cups (280g) shredded

carrots, ¼ cup (30g) diced

cauliflower florets, 1 pound (454g)

celery, 3½ ounces (100g)

chives, 1 small bunch

collard leaves, 4 large

dill, 1 small bunch

garlic, 9 cloves (or 3 tablespoons jarred minced garlic)

Hass avocados, 2 medium (about 7½ ounces/212g each)

lemon, 1

limes, 2

onions, 2 small (about 2½ ounces/70g each)

parsley, 1 bunch

Roma tomato, 1 large (about 3½ ounces/100g)

scallions, 1 bunch

zucchini noodles, 8 ounces (225g)

Freezer Items:

chopped spinach, 6 ounces (170g)

riced cauliflower, 12 ounces (340g)

Refrigerated Items:

dairy-free buttery spread, 2 tablespoons, or 2 additional tablespoons olive oil

extra-firm tofu, 14-ounce (397-g) block

Kalamata olives, 2 ounces (56g)

nondairy milk of choice, ¾ cup (180ml)

nondairy yogurt, ½ cup (120ml)

plant-based ground, 2 (1-pound/454-g) packages

prepared yellow mustard, 1 tablespoon

salsa, 2 tablespoons

shirataki (konjac/"miracle") noodles,
2 (8-ounce/225-g) packages
tempeh, 2 (8-ounce/225-g) packages

Pantry Items:

allulose syrup or other sugar-free syrup of
choice, ½ cup (120ml), or 2 additional
tablespoons granulated sweetener
apple cider vinegar, 1 teaspoon
baking powder, ½ teaspoon
baking soda, ¼ teaspoon
canned pumpkin, ¼ cup plus 2 tablespoons
(90g)
chili paste, Sriracha sauce, or other hot
sauce, 1 teaspoon
coconut flour, ¼ cup plus 2 tablespoons
(42g)
coconut oil, 2 tablespoons
extra-virgin olive oil, 12 ounces (720ml)
freeze-dried strawberries, ½ cup (5g)
granulated sweetener, 2 tablespoons
liquid stevia, ⅛ teaspoon
lupin flour, ½ cup (60g)
nutritional yeast, ¼ cup (16g)
psyllium husks, 1 tablespoon
red wine vinegar, 3 tablespoons
sugar-free maple syrup, 2 tablespoons
sugar-free vanilla protein powder,
2 tablespoons
tamari, low sodium, ¼ cup plus
2 tablespoons (90ml)
unsweetened chocolate chips, ½ cup (120g)
vanilla extract, 2 teaspoons

Nuts & Seeds:

almond butter, ½ cup (128g)
almonds, 1 cup (120g)
ground flaxseed, 6 ounces (170g)
hulled hemp seeds, 5 ounces (140g)
peanut butter, unsweetened, ¾ cup plus
2 tablespoons (224g)
peanuts, ½ cup (60g)
pumpkin seeds (pepitas), ½ cup (60g)
sesame seeds, ½ cup (80g)
walnuts, raw, 1 cup (120g)

Dried Herbs & Spices:

black pepper
chili powder
Chinese five-spice powder
dried oregano leaves
dried thyme leaves
ginger powder
granulated garlic
Greek seasoning (page 148, or store-
bought)
pumpkin pie spice
red pepper flakes
salt
smoked paprika
taco seasoning
white pepper (optional, or use black pepper)

> **NOTE**
>
> The shopping lists do not include optional
> ingredients or suggested toppings or
> garnishes.

Week 2: ~30g Net Carbs Daily

	Breakfast	Lunch	
Day 1	**No-Bake White Chocolate–Raspberry Bars (page 258) (x2)**	**Shepherd's Pie (page 158)**	
Day 2	No-Bake White Chocolate–Raspberry Bars (x2)	Green Goddess Bowl	
Day 3	**Overnight "N'Oats" (page 104)**	Super Crispy Baked Tofu Rainbow Veggie Pilaf (x2) + 1 tablespoon olive oil	
Day 4	**Raspberry Power Smoothie (page 112)**	Cabbage Noodle Chow Mein + Basic Baked Tofu	
Day 5	Overnight "N'Oats" (page 104)	**Broccoli Noodle Bowl with Peanut Sauce (page 168)**	
Day 6	**Greek Stuffed Pepper (page 148)** **Roasted Lemon-Pepper Asparagus (page 220)**	Broccoli Noodle Bowl with Peanut Sauce	
Day 7	**Overnight "N'Oats" (page 104)**	Basic Baked Tofu Sesame-Garlic Kale (x2)	

Dinner	Snacks	Nutrition
Green Goddess Bowl (page 162)	PB&J Muffin ½ cup (60g) almonds	**Calories:** 1680 **Fat:** 138g **Protein:** 73g **Total Carbs:** 67.7g **Net Carbs:** 28.8g
Super Crispy Baked Tofu (page 172) (x2) **Rainbow Veggie Pilaf (page 214) +** 1½ teaspoons olive oil	½ cup (60g) almonds	**Calories:** 1693 **Fat:** 138.9g **Protein:** 74g **Total Carbs:** 60.7g **Net Carbs:** 28.9g
Cabbage Noodle Chow Mein + Basic Baked Tofu	No-Bake White Chocolate–Raspberry Bars (x2) ¼ cup (30g) almonds	**Calories:** 1681 **Fat:** 135g **Protein:** 74.4g **Total Carbs:** 62.3g **Net Carbs:** 29.7g
Super Crispy Baked Tofu Rainbow Veggie Pilaf (x2) + 1 tablespoon olive oil	No-Bake White Chocolate–Raspberry Bars (x2)	**Calories:** 1698 **Fat:** 137.2g **Protein:** 70.6g **Total Carbs:** 65.2g **Net Carbs:** 31.6g
Basic Baked Tofu (page 170) Rainbow Veggie Pilaf + Chimichurri	1 cup (100g) celery sticks + Pantry Peanut Sauce Dark Chocolate Truffles (x4)	**Calories:** 1602 **Fat:** 122.6g **Protein:** 75.8g **Total Carbs:** 82.9g **Net Carbs:** 31.7g
Basic Baked Tofu (x2) **Sesame-Garlic Kale (page 212) (x2)**	2 ounces (56g) Kalamata olives Dark Chocolate Truffles (x2)	**Calories:** 1560 **Fat:** 125.2g **Protein:** 70.4g **Total Carbs:** 69.1g **Net Carbs:** 31.4g
Greek Stuffed Pepper Roasted Lemon-Pepper Asparagus (x2)	1 cup (100g) celery sticks + Pantry Peanut Sauce ½ cup (60g) almonds Dark Chocolate Truffles (x2)	**Calories:** 1685 **Fat:** 135g **Protein:** 74.2g **Total Carbs:** 75g **Net Carbs:** 30g

Week 2 Notes

Day 1: Use the leftover Green Goddess Dressing and PB&J Muffin from Week 1.

Days 3 & 4: Use the leftover Cabbage Noodle Chow Mein and Basic Baked Tofu from Week 1.

Day 4: Raspberry Power Smoothie is a variation of the Raspberry-Beet Power Smoothie (page 112).

Day 5: Use the leftover Chimichurri, Pantry Peanut Sauce, and Dark Chocolate Truffles from Week 1.

Week 2 Ingredients

Produce:

asparagus, 1 bunch (about 1 pound/454g)
baby spinach, 2 cups (60g)
broccoli, 1 medium head
carrot, 5 ounces (140g)
cauliflower florets, 1 pound (454g)
celery sticks, 3½ cups (350g)
cucumber, 1 medium (about 7 ounces/ 200g)
edamame, shelled, 1 cup (155g)
garlic, 3 cloves (or 1 tablespoon jarred minced garlic)
Hass avocado, 1 medium (about 7½ ounces/ 212g)
kale, 6 cups (125g) chopped
lemon, 1
onion, ½ small (about 1¼ ounces/35g)
radishes, 4 ounces (112g)
zucchini noodles, 8 ounces (225g)

Produce Left Over from Week 1:

bell pepper, ½ small (about 1¼ ounces/35g)
chives
parsley
scallions

Freezer Items:

raspberries, ⅔ cup (60g)
riced cauliflower, 12 ounces (340g)

Refrigerated Items:

cream cheese, nondairy or dairy, ½ cup (128g)
dairy-free buttery spread, 2 tablespoons, or 2 additional tablespoons olive oil
extra-firm tofu, 2 (14-ounce/397-g) blocks
Kalamata olives, 4 ounces (112g)
nondairy milk of choice, 3¼ cups (780ml)
plant-based ground, 1-pound (454-g) package

Pantry Items:

black soybean noodles, 2 ounces (56g)

cacao butter or coconut oil, ½ cup (112g)

coconut flour, ¼ cup plus 2 tablespoons
    (42g)

extra-virgin olive oil, ½ cup plus
    1 tablespoon (135ml)

freeze-dried raspberries or strawberries,
    ½ cup (10g)

liquid stevia, ⅛ teaspoon

MCT oil or coconut oil, 1 tablespoon

nutritional yeast, ¼ cup (16g)

toasted sesame oil, 2 ounces (60ml)

vanilla protein powder, ⅞ cup (150g)

vegetable broth, ½ cup (120ml)

Nuts & Seeds:

almonds, 1¾ cups (210g)

ground flaxseed, ¼ cup plus 2 tablespoons
    (42g)

hulled hemp seeds, ¾ cup (120g)

peanuts, ½ cup (60g)

sesame seeds, 2 tablespoons

sunflower seeds, ½ cup (60g)

Dried Herbs & Spices:

black pepper

granulated garlic

ground cinnamon

red pepper flakes

salt

Week 3: ~30g Net Carbs Daily (Soy-Free)

	Breakfast	Lunch	
Day 1	**Falafel Waffle (page 98) + Chimichurri (page 242)**	**Hemp Seed Tabbouleh (page 134)**	
Day 2	Falafel Waffle + Chimichurri	Empanada-Inspired Salad + Chimichurri	
Day 3	**Overnight "N'Oats" (page 104)**	Hemp Seed Tabbouleh	
Day 4	**Raspberry Power Smoothie (page 112)**	Hemp Seed Tabbouleh	
Day 5	**Overnight "N'Oats" (page 104)**	Mushroom "Meatballs" Pistachio Pesto Brussels Sprouts	
Day 6	**Raspberry Mini Smoothie Bowl (page 114)**	**Broccoli Tots (page 228) (x2) +** Pistachio Parsley Pesto Sesame-Garlic Kale	
Day 7	Raspberry Mini Smoothie Bowl	Broccoli Tots (x2) + Pistachio Parsley Pesto Sesame-Garlic Kale	

Dinner	Snacks	Nutrition
Empanada-Inspired Salad (page 151) + Chimichurri	1 cup (100g) celery sticks + 2 tablespoons peanut butter ¼ cup (30g) almonds	Calories: 1553 Fat: 122.2g Protein: 70.4g Total Carbs: 66.8g Net Carbs: 28.9g
Mushroom "Meatballs" (page 178) **Pistachio Pesto Brussels Sprouts (page 224)**	½ cup (60g) almonds	Calories: 1651 Fat: 133.7g Protein: 72.5g Total Carbs: 70.8g Net Carbs: 29.9g
Mushroom "Meatballs" Pistachio Pesto Brussels Sprouts	½ cup (50g) celery sticks + 1 tablespoon peanut butter ½ cup (60g) almonds	Calories: 1553 Fat: 125.1g Protein: 67.8g Total Carbs: 66.1g Net Carbs: 29.7g
Lupin Spinach Fritters (page 234) (x2) + Pistachio Parsley Pesto	½ cup (50g) celery sticks + 1 tablespoon peanut butter ½ cup (60g) almonds	Calories: 1614 Fat: 125.1g Protein: 69.4g Total Carbs: 79.7g Net Carbs: 29.4g
Lupin Spinach Fritters + Pistachio Parsley Pesto **Sesame-Garlic Kale (page 212)**	1 cup (100g) celery sticks + 2 tablespoons peanut butter	Calories: 1680 Fat: 134.5g Protein: 71.3g Total Carbs: 75.6g Net Carbs: 29.5g
Korma-Inspired Cauliflower Bake (page 160)	**Basic Protein Shake*** ½ cup (56g) macadamia nuts	Calories: 1618 Fat: 132.4g Protein: 73.2g Total Carbs: 58.9g Net Carbs: 31.5g
Korma-Inspired Cauliflower Bake	**Basic Protein Shake*** ½ cup (56g) macadamia nuts	Calories: 1618 Fat: 132.4g Protein: 73.2g Total Carbs: 58.9g Net Carbs: 31.5g

Week 3 Notes

Day 1: Yes, I paired the waffle with Chimichurri—it's really good! You could also make the yogurt sauce, though.

If you followed Weeks 1 and 2, you will have a leftover half package of plant-based ground.

Day 2: Freeze 3 servings of Pistachio Parsley Pesto for Week 4.

Day 4: Raspberry Power Smoothie is a variation of the Raspberry-Beet Power Smoothie (page 112).

Day 6: Raspberry Mini Smoothie Bowls are a variation of the Blackberry Yogurt Smoothie Bowl (page 114).

Divide the batch of tots in half for a meal-sized portion.

The ginger root piece is enough for both the Korma-Inspired Cauliflower Bake and the Pantry Peanut Sauce in Week 4.

Set aside half of the Korma-Inspired Cauliflower Bake for Week 4.

*Basic Protein Shake = 1 scoop of your favorite sugar-free protein powder + 8 ounces (240ml) water or nondairy milk.

Week 3 Ingredients

Produce:

baby greens, 4 cups (120g)

baby spinach, 1 lightly packed cup (30g)

bell pepper, red, ½ small (about 1¼ ounces/ 35g)

broccoli florets, 3 cups (210g)

Brussels sprouts, shaved, 12 ounces (340g)

carrot, 1 small (about 1¾ ounces/50g)

cauliflower florets, 1 pound (454g)

celery sticks, 3 cups (300g)

cucumber, 1 medium (about 8 ounces/ 225g)

dill, 1 small bunch

garlic, 15 cloves (or 5 tablespoons jarred minced garlic)

ginger, 2-inch (5-cm) knob

grape tomatoes, 8 ounces (225g)

kale, 6 cups (125g) chopped

lemons, 1½

mint, 1 small bunch

mushrooms, button or cremini, 8 ounces (225g)

onion, 1 small (about 2½ ounces/70g)
parsley, 2 large bunches
scallions, 1 bunch

Freezer Items:

chopped spinach, 8 ounces (225g)
raspberries, 1 cup (90g)
riced cauliflower, 3½ ounces (100g)

Refrigerated Items:

coconut yogurt, 1 cup (240ml)
nondairy milk of choice, 2½ cups (600ml)*
plant-based ground, 8 ounces (225g)
prepared yellow mustard, 1 tablespoon

*Add 2 cups (480ml) nondairy milk if using milk instead of water in the Basic Protein Shake.

Pantry Items:

coconut flour, ¼ cup (28g)
coconut milk, canned full-fat, ⅔ cup (160ml)
extra-virgin olive oil, 1¼ cups plus 1 tablespoon (315ml)
liquid stevia, ¼ teaspoon
lupin flour, 1 cup (120g)
MCT oil or coconut oil, 1 tablespoon
nutritional yeast, ¾ cup (48g)
psyllium husks, ¼ cup (20g)
red wine vinegar, 3 tablespoons
toasted sesame oil, 2 tablespoons
tomato paste, 1 tablespoon
vanilla protein powder, ½ cup (60g)

Nuts & Seeds:

almonds, 1¾ cups (210g)
chia seeds, 1 teaspoon
ground flaxseed, ¼ cup plus 1 teaspoon (30g)
hulled hemp seeds, 2 cups plus 2 tablespoons plus 1 teaspoon (345g)
macadamia nuts, 1 cup (112g)
peanut butter, unsweetened, ¼ cup plus 2 tablespoons (96g)
pistachios, shelled raw, ½ cup plus 2 tablespoons (75g)
sesame seeds, 1 tablespoon
tahini, ½ cup plus 2 tablespoons (150ml)

Dried Herbs & Spices:

black pepper
chili powder
dehydrated onion flakes
dried oregano leaves
dried parsley
dried thyme leaves
garam masala
granulated garlic
ground cinnamon
ground cumin
red pepper flakes
salt
smoked paprika

Week 4: ~30g Net Carbs Daily (Soy-Free)

	Breakfast	Lunch	
Day 1	**Pumpkin Spice Breakfast Bars (page 110) (x2)**	Korma-Inspired Cauliflower Bake	
Day 2	**Overnight "N'Oats" (page 104)**	Korma-Inspired Cauliflower Bake	
Day 3	Pumpkin Spice Breakfast Bars (x2) + 1 tablespoon peanut butter	Garlic Sesame "Meatballs" 1 cup (100g) broccoli florets + 1½ teaspoons olive oil	
Day 4	**Raspberry Power Smoothie (page 112)**	Shepherd's Pie	
Day 5	**Overnight "N'Oats" (page 104)**	Pistachio Pesto Flatbread Roasted Lemon-Pepper Asparagus	
Day 6	**Crunchy Peanut Butter Muffins (page 107) (x2)**	Shepherd's Pie	
Day 7	Crunchy Peanut Butter Muffins (x3)	Peanutty Veggie Noodle Bowl	

Dinner	Snacks	Nutrition
Garlic Sesame "Meatballs" (page 178) **Sesame-Garlic Kale (page 212)**	1 cup (100g) celery sticks + **Raw Muhammara (page 210)** ¼ cup (28g) macadamia nuts	**Calories:** 1606 **Fat:** 131.1g **Protein:** 73g **Total Carbs:** 58.9g **Net Carbs:** 30g
Garlic Sesame "Meatballs" 1 cup (100g) broccoli florets + 1½ teaspoons olive oil	Pumpkin Spice Breakfast Bars (x2) 1 cup (100g) celery sticks + Raw Muhammara	**Calories:** 1597 **Fat:** 124.3g **Protein:** 73.5g **Total Carbs:** 69.9g **Net Carbs:** 31.8g
Shepherd's Pie (page 158)	1 cup (100g) celery sticks + Raw Muhammara ½ cup (60g) almonds	**Calories:** 1667 **Fat:** 137.2g **Protein:** 72.5g **Total Carbs:** 64.1g **Net Carbs:** 30.5g
Pistachio Pesto Flatbread (page 140) (x2)	Pumpkin Spice Breakfast Bars (x2) ¼ cup (28g) macadamia nuts	**Calories:** 1650 **Fat:** 129g **Protein:** 73g **Total Carbs:** 64.1g **Net Carbs:** 30.5g
Shepherd's Pie	1 cup (100g) celery sticks + Raw Muhammara (x2) Pumpkin Spice Breakfast Bar + 1 tablespoon peanut butter	**Calories:** 1597 **Fat:** 125.7g **Protein:** 73.3g **Total Carbs:** 68.7g **Net Carbs:** 30.7g
Peanutty Veggie Noodle Bowl (page 164)	**Basic Protein Shake*** 1 cup (100g) celery sticks + Raw Muhammara ¼ cup (28g) macadamia nuts	**Calories:** 1577 **Fat:** 126g **Protein:** 77.4g **Total Carbs:** 68.4g **Net Carbs:** 30.6g
Pistachio Pesto Flatbread Roasted Lemon-Pepper Asparagus	**Basic Protein Shake*** ¼ cup (28g) macadamia nuts	**Calories:** 1656 **Fat:** 133.6g **Protein:** 68.8g **Total Carbs:** 82.4g **Net Carbs:** 32.4g

Week 4 Notes

Day 1: Garlic Sesame "Meatballs" are a variation of the Mushroom "Meatballs" (page 178).

Freeze half of the Raw Muhammara for later in the week.

Day 2: Sauté 2 cups (200g) of broccoli florets with 1 tablespoon of olive oil until tender. Season with salt and pepper to taste. Serve half today and half on Day 3.

Day 3: I make a little sandwich out of the peanut butter and breakfast bars and eat it with my coffee.

Day 4: Pistachio Pesto Flatbread is a variation of the Veggie Flatbreads (page 140). Use the leftover Pistachio Parsley Pesto from Week 3.

Day 5: Use the Roasted Lemon-Pepper Asparagus left over from making the Pistachio Pesto Flatbread.

Day 6: Crunchy Peanut Butter Muffins are a variation of the PB&J Muffins (page 106).

Make a half batch of the Pantry Peanut Sauce (using coconut aminos in place of tamari to make it soy-free). You will have 1 serving (2 tablespoons) left over at the end of the week.

*Basic Protein Shake = 1 scoop of your favorite sugar-free protein powder + 8 ounces (240ml) water or nondairy milk.

Week 4 Ingredients

Produce:

asparagus, 1 bunch (about 1 pound/454g)
baby spinach, 1 lightly packed cup (30g)
bell pepper, red, 1 large (about 6 ounces/ 170g)
broccoli florets, 2 cups (200g)
carrots, 2 small (about 3½ ounces/100g)
cauliflower florets, 2 pounds (908g)
celery sticks, 5½ cups (550g)
chives, 1 small bunch
garlic, 11 cloves (or 3 tablespoons plus 2 teaspoons jarred minced garlic)
kale, 6 cups (125g) chopped
lemon, 1
lime, 1

mushrooms, button or cremini, 8 ounces (225g)
spinach, 1 lightly packed cup (30g)
summer squash or zucchini, 2 medium (about 7 ounces/200g each)
zucchini noodles, 8 ounces (225g)

Produce Left Over from Week 3:

ginger root
onion, ½ small (about 1¼ ounces/35g)
scallions

Freezer Items:

raspberries, ⅔ cup (60g)

Refrigerated Items:

dairy-free buttery spread, 2 tablespoons, or 2 additional tablespoons olive oil
nondairy milk of choice, 2½ cups (600ml)*
plant-based ground, 1-pound (454-g) package

*Add 2 cups (480ml) of nondairy milk if using milk instead of water in the Basic Protein Shake.

Pantry Items:

apple cider vinegar, 1 teaspoon
baking powder, ½ teaspoon
baking soda, ¼ teaspoon
canned pumpkin, ¼ cup plus 2 tablespoons (90g)
chili paste, Sriracha sauce, or other hot sauce, ½ teaspoon
coconut aminos, 1½ teaspoons
coconut flour, ½ cup (56g)
coconut milk, canned full-fat, ⅔ cup (160ml)

coconut oil, 2 tablespoons
extra-virgin olive oil, ¼ cup plus 2 tablespoons
granulated sweetener, 2 tablespoons
liquid stevia, ¼ teaspoon
MCT oil or coconut oil, 1 tablespoon
nutritional yeast, ½ cup (32g)
psyllium husks, ¼ cup plus 1 tablespoon (25g)
toasted sesame oil, 3 tablespoons
tomato paste, 1 tablespoon
vanilla extract, 2 teaspoons
vanilla protein powder, ¾ cup (90g)

Nuts & Seeds:

almonds, ½ cup (60g)
ground flaxseed, ½ cup (56g)
hulled hemp seeds, 2 cups plus 2 tablespoons (340g)
macadamia nuts, 1 cup (112g)
peanut butter, unsweetened, ¾ cup (192g)
peanuts, ½ cup plus 2 tablespoons (75g)
pumpkin seeds (pepitas), ¼ cup (30g)
sesame seeds, ½ cup plus 3 tablespoons (110g)
tahini, ½ cup (128g)
walnuts, raw, 1 cup (120g)

Dried Herbs & Spices:

black pepper
garam masala
granulated garlic
ground cinnamon
ground cumin
pumpkin pie spice
red pepper flakes
salt
smoked paprika

Week 1: ~45g Net Carbs Daily

	Breakfast	Lunch	
Day 1	**Pizza Muffins (page 108) (x2)** **Cabbage & Kale Hash (page 100)**	**Waldorf Kale Salad (page 132) (x2)**	
Day 2	Pizza Muffins (x2) Cabbage & Kale Hash	Thai-Inspired Cauliflower Coconut Curry + Super Crispy Baked Tofu	
Day 3	Pumpkin Spice Breakfast Bars (x3)	Cabbage & Kale Hash (x2)	
Day 4	**Blackberry Yogurt Smoothie Bowl (page 114)**	Shepherd's Pie Balsamic Beets & Greens	
Day 5	**Raspberry-Beet Power Smoothie (page 112)**	Mushroom Stroganoff (x2)	
Day 6	**Falafel Waffle (page 98)** + Yogurt Dill Sauce	Shepherd's Pie Balsamic Beets & Greens	
Day 7	Falafel Waffle + Yogurt Dill Sauce	Korma-Inspired Cauliflower Bake	

	Dinner	Snacks	Nutrition
	Thai-Inspired Cauliflower Coconut Curry (page 144) + Super Crispy Baked Tofu (page 172)	**Pumpkin Spice Breakfast Bars (page 110) (x2)** 1 cup (100g) celery sticks + 2 tablespoons peanut butter	**Calories:** 1883 **Fat:** 146.9g **Protein:** 77.8g **Total Carbs:** 92.9g **Net Carbs:** 42.8g
	Shepherd's Pie (page 158) **Balsamic Beets & Greens (page 216)**	Pumpkin Spice Breakfast Bars (x2) + 1 tablespoon peanut butter	**Calories:** 1704 **Fat:** 129.4g **Protein:** 83g **Total Carbs:** 78.9g **Net Carbs:** 40.6g
	Thai-Inspired Cauliflower Coconut Curry (x2) + Super Crispy Baked Tofu (x2)	¼ cup (28g) macadamia nuts	**Calories:** 1842 **Fat:** 146.7g **Protein:** 77.2g **Total Carbs:** 72.6g **Net Carbs:** 39.7g
	Mushroom Stroganoff (page 146) (x2)	Pumpkin Spice Breakfast Bars (x2) ¼ cup (28g) macadamia nuts	**Calories:** 1727 **Fat:** 138g **Protein:** 74.5g **Total Carbs:** 72.6g **Net Carbs:** 40.3g
	Shepherd's Pie Balsamic Beets & Greens	**Lupin Spinach Fritters (page 234) (x1.5) + Yogurt Dill Sauce (page 240)** ½ cup (56g) macadamia nuts	**Calories:** 1756 **Fat:** 140.7g **Protein:** 69.8g **Total Carbs:** 87.4g **Net Carbs:** 40.4g
	Korma-Inspired Cauliflower Bake (page 160)	Lupin Spinach Fritters (x1.5) + Yogurt Dill Sauce ½ cup (56g) macadamia nuts	**Calories:** 1744 **Fat:** 137.4g **Protein:** 77.4g **Total Carbs:** 91.1g **Net Carbs:** 41.7g
	Peanutty Veggie Noodle Bowl (page 164)	**Tofu Fries (page 232) + Pantry Peanut Sauce (page 243)** ½ cup (56g) macadamia nuts	**Calories:** 1734 **Fat:** 139.3g **Protein:** 79.3g **Total Carbs:** 19.3g **Net Carbs:** 39.1g

Week 1 Notes

Days 1 & 2: Spread the peanut butter on one of the breakfast bars and place the other on top to make a little snack sandwich.

Day 2: Freeze the remainder of the Balsamic Vinaigrette for Week 3.

Day 5: If you don't love the idea of beets in a smoothie, you can replace them with more raspberries (see the Raspberry Power Smoothie variation on page 112).

Day 7: Make the PB&J Muffins tonight for breakfast tomorrow (Day 1 of Week 2), unless you are a morning person!

Week 1 Ingredients

Produce:

baby spinach, 1 lightly packed cup (30g)

beet greens, 2 cups (about 3 ounces/85g)

beets, 1 medium bunch (about 8 ounces/ 225g)

bell pepper, yellow, orange, or red, 1 medium (about 4 ounces/120g)

bell pepper, red, 1 small (about 2½ ounces/ 70g)

carrots, 2 small (about 1¾ ounces/ 50g each)

cauliflower, 2 large heads (about 3¼ pounds/1.5kg)*

celery sticks, 2½ cups (250g)

chives, 1 small bunch

dill, 1 bunch

garlic, 9 cloves (or 3 tablespoons jarred minced garlic)

ginger, 2-inch (5-cm) piece

green cabbage, ¼ small head (about 7 ounces/200g)

jicama, 4 ounces (112g)

kale, 1 large bunch

lemon, 1

lime, 1

mushrooms, button or cremini, 1 pound (454g)

onion, 1 small (about 2½ ounces/70g)

scallions, 1 bunch

shallot, 1 small

spaghetti squash, ½ small (about 10½ ounces/300g)

zucchini, 1 small (about 4¼ ounces/120g)

zucchini noodles, 8 ounces (225g)

*You can also buy frozen cauliflower for these recipes!

Freezer Items:

blackberries, ⅓ cup (50g)

chopped spinach, 8 ounces (225g)

raspberries, ⅓ cup (30g)

riced cauliflower, ½ cup (56g)

Refrigerated Items:

chili paste, Sriracha sauce, or other hot
   sauce, 1 teaspoon
coconut yogurt, 2 cups (480ml)
dairy-free buttery spread, 2 tablespoons, or
   2 additional tablespoons olive oil
Dijon mustard, 2 tablespoons
extra-firm tofu, 2 (14-ounce/397-g) blocks
pea milk or other nondairy milk of choice,
   1 cup (240ml)
plant-based ground, 1-pound (454-g)
   package
prepared yellow mustard, 1 tablespoon

Pantry Items:

apple cider vinegar, 3 tablespoons
baking powder, 1 teaspoon
balsamic vinegar, ¼ cup (60ml)
canned pumpkin, ¼ cup plus 2 tablespoons
   (90g)
coconut cream, ½ cup (120ml)
coconut flour, 2 tablespoons
coconut milk, full-fat, 2 (13.5-ounce/
   397-g) cans
extra-virgin olive oil, 1¾ cups (420ml)
liquid stevia, ⅜ teaspoon
lupin flour, 1¼ cups (150g)
MCT oil or coconut oil, 1 tablespoon
nutritional yeast, ¾ cup (48g)
psyllium husks, 2 tablespoons plus
   1 teaspoon
tamari, low-sodium, 1 tablespoon
Thai red curry paste, 2 tablespoons
tomato paste, 1 tablespoon
tomato sauce, low-sugar, ½ cup (120ml)
vanilla extract, 1 teaspoon
vanilla protein powder, ¼ cup (30g)

Nuts & Seeds:

chia seeds, 1 teaspoon
ground flaxseed, 2 tablespoons plus
   1 teaspoon
hulled hemp seeds, 1½ cups plus
   3 tablespoons (270g)
macadamia nuts, 8 ounces (225g)
peanut butter, ½ cup plus 3 tablespoons
   (175g)
peanuts, chopped, ½ cup (60g)
pumpkin seeds (pepitas), ¼ cup (30g)
sesame seeds, ½ cup (80g)
tahini, ¼ cup (60ml)
walnuts, raw, ½ cup (60g)

Dried Herbs & Spices:

black pepper
dehydrated onion flakes
dried oregano leaves
dried parsley
dried thyme leaves
garam masala
garlic powder
ginger powder
granulated garlic
ground cinnamon
ground cumin
paprika
pumpkin pie spice
red pepper flakes
salt
smoked paprika
white pepper

Week 2: ~45g Net Carbs Daily

	Breakfast	Lunch	
Day 1	**PB&J Muffins (page 106) (x2)**	**Peanutty Veggie Noodle Bowl (page 164)**	
Day 2	PB&J Muffins (x3)	Korma-Inspired Cauliflower Bake Rainbow Veggie Pilaf	
Day 3	**Raspberry Mini Smoothie Bowl (page 114)**	Empanada-Inspired Collard Wraps + Chimichurri Rainbow Veggie Pilaf (x2)	
Day 4	Raspberry Mini Smoothie Bowl	Avocado & Grapefruit Salad (x2) + Basic Baked Tofu (x2)	
Day 5	**Overnight "N'Oats" (page 104)**	**Lemony Noodles with Peas & Edamame (page 154)**	
Day 6	**Crunchy Peanut Butter Muffins (page 107) (x2)**	Moroccan-Inspired Butternut Squash Stew (x2) + Cumin Spice "Meatballs"	
Day 7	Crunchy Peanut Butter Muffins (x3)	Lemony Noodles with Peas & Edamame	

Dinner	Snacks	Nutrition
Korma-Inspired Cauliflower Bake (page 160) **Rainbow Veggie Pilaf (page 214)**	**Tofu Fries (page 232)** + Pantry Peanut Sauce **Dark Chocolate Truffles (page 252) (x2)**	**Calories:** 1732 **Fat:** 135.9g **Protein:** 75.8g **Total Carbs:** 92.4g **Net Carbs:** 42g
Empanada-Inspired Collard Wraps (page 150) + Chimichurri (page 242) Rainbow Veggie Pilaf	Tofu Fries + Chimichurri	**Calories:** 1861 **Fat:** 148.9g **Protein:** 79.7g **Total Carbs:** 88.6g **Net Carbs:** 39.2g
Avocado & Grapefruit Salad (page 130) (x2) + Basic Baked Tofu (page 170) (x2)	1 cup (100g) celery sticks + Pantry Peanut Sauce Dark Chocolate Truffles (x2)	**Calories:** 1864 **Fat:** 145.6g **Protein:** 83.5g **Total Carbs:** 89.5g **Net Carbs:** 41.5g
Moroccan-Inspired Butternut Squash Stew (page 142) Rainbow Veggie Pilaf (x2)	1 cup (100g) celery sticks + Pantry Peanut Sauce ¼ cup (28g) macadamia nuts Dark Chocolate Truffles (x2)	**Calories:** 1807 **Fat:** 142.3g **Protein:** 70.4g **Total Carbs:** 93.2g **Net Carbs:** 44.2g
Moroccan-Inspired Butternut Squash Stew (x2) + **Cumin Spice "Meatballs" (page 178)**	¼ cup (28g) macadamia nuts 1 cup (100g) celery sticks + 2 tablespoons peanut butter Dark Chocolate Truffles (x2)	**Calories:** 1784 **Fat:** 134.9g **Protein:** 75.3g **Total Carbs:** 91.9g **Net Carbs:** 43.7g
Cabbage Noodle Chow Mein (page 152) (x2) + Basic Baked Tofu (page 170) (x2)	¼ cup (28g) macadamia nuts	**Calories:** 1884 **Fat:** 148.7g **Protein:** 70.9g **Total Carbs:** 93.7g **Net Carbs:** 46.2g
Cabbage Noodle Chow Mein (x2) + Basic Baked Tofu (x2)	1 cup (100g) sliced cucumbers + Chimichurri	**Calories:** 1824 **Fat:** 142.8g **Protein:** 69.5g **Total Carbs:** 98.1g **Net Carbs:** 45g

Week 2 Notes

Day 2: Freeze half the package of plant-based ground and two servings of Chimichurri for Week 3.

Day 3: Raspberry Mini Smoothie Bowls are a variation of the Blackberry Yogurt Smoothie Bowl (page 114).

Day 5: Cumin Spice "Meatballs" are a variation of the Mushroom "Meatballs" (page 178).

Day 6: Crunchy Peanut Butter Muffins are a variation of the PB&J Muffins (page 106).

Week 2 Ingredients

Produce:

bell pepper, red, ½ small (about 1¼ ounces/ 35g)

butternut squash, 1 cup (200g) cubed

cabbage, shredded, 4 cups (280g)

carrot, 1 small (about 1¾ ounces/50g)

cauliflower florets, 1 pound (454g)

celery sticks, 3½ cups (350g)

collard leaves, 4 large

cucumbers, 1 cup sliced (100g)

garlic, 9 cloves (or 3 tablespoons jarred minced garlic)

ginger, 1-inch (2.5-cm) piece

grapefruit sections, ½ cup (115g)

Hass avocados, 2 medium (about 7½ ounces/212g each)

kale, 6 cups (125g) chopped

lemon, 1

lime, 1

mushrooms, button or cremini, 8 ounces (225g)

onion, 1 small (about 2½ ounces/70g)

parsley, 1 large bunch

riced broccoli, 4 ounces (112g)

riced carrots, 4 ounces (112g)

riced radishes, 4 ounces (112g)

scallions, 2

shallot, 1 small

zucchini noodles, 8 ounces (225g)

Freezer Items:

edamame, shelled, ½ cup (80g)

peas, ¼ cup (40g)

raspberries, ⅓ cup (50g)

riced cauliflower, 18 ounces (500g)

Refrigerated Items:

coconut yogurt, ½ cup (120ml)

extra-firm tofu, 3 (14-ounce/397-g) blocks

nondairy milk of choice, ¾ cup (180ml)

plant-based ground, 8 ounces (225g)

Pantry Items:

allulose syrup or other sugar-free syrup,
 ¼ cup (60ml), or 2 additional tablespoons
 granulated sweetener

apple cider vinegar, 2 teaspoons

baking powder, 1 teaspoon

baking soda, ½ teaspoon

chili paste, Sriracha sauce, or other hot
 sauce, 1 teaspoon

coconut flour, ½ cup plus 2 tablespoons
 (70g)

coconut milk, canned full-fat, ⅔ cup
 (160ml)

coconut oil, ¼ cup (60ml)

diced tomatoes, canned, 1 cup (240ml)

extra-virgin olive oil, 1½ cups (360ml)

freeze-dried strawberries, ½ cup (5g)

granulated sweetener, ¼ cup (48g)

liquid stevia, ⅛ teaspoon

lupini beans, jarred (packed in brine), 1 cup
 (170g)

nutritional yeast, ¼ cup (16g)

psyllium husks, 1 tablespoon

red wine vinegar, 3 tablespoons

shirataki noodles, 2 (8-ounce/225-g)
 packages

tamari, low-sodium, ¼ cup (60ml)

tomato paste, 1 tablespoon

unsweetened chocolate chips, ¼ cup (60g)

vanilla extract, 2 teaspoons

vanilla protein powder, ¼ cup plus
 2 tablespoons (45g)

vegetable broth, 1½ cups (360ml)

Nuts & Seeds:

almond butter, ¼ cup (64g)

almonds, sliced, ¼ cup (30g)

chia seeds, 1 teaspoon

ground flaxseed, 6 tablespoons plus
 1 teaspoon (63g)

hulled hemp seeds, 1¼ cups plus
 2 tablespoons plus 1 teaspoon (223g)

macadamia nuts, ¾ cup (84g)

peanut butter, 1¼ cups (320g)

peanuts, ½ cup plus 2 tablespoons (75g)

sunflower seeds, ½ cup (60g)

tahini, ¼ cup (60ml)

Dried Herbs & Spices:

black pepper

chili powder

Chinese five-spice powder

dehydrated onion flakes

dried oregano leaves

dried parsley

dried thyme leaves

garam masala

garlic powder

ginger powder

granulated garlic

ground cinnamon

ground cumin

ras el hanout

red pepper flakes

salt

smoked paprika

white pepper

Week 3: ~45g Net Carbs Daily (Soy-Free)

	Breakfast	Lunch	
Day 1	**No-Bake White Chocolate–Raspberry Bars (page 258) (x2)**	**Hemp Seed Tabbouleh (page 134)**	
Day 2	**Pumpkin Spice Breakfast Bars (page 110) (x2)** ¾ cup (180ml) coconut yogurt	Empanada-Inspired Salad + Chimichurri	
Day 3	No-Bake White Chocolate–Raspberry Bars (x2)	Hemp Seed Tabbouleh	
Day 4	Pumpkin Spice Breakfast Bars (x3) ¾ cup (180ml) coconut yogurt	Hemp Seed Tabbouleh	
Day 5	**Raspberry-Beet Power Smoothie (page 112)**	Lupin Spinach Fritters + Yogurt Dill Sauce Balsamic Beets & Greens (x2)	
Day 6	**Shakshuka (page 102)**	Korma-Inspired Cauliflower Bake	
Day 7	Shakshuka	Cumin Spice "Meatballs" Pumpkin Spice Mashed Butternut Squash (x2)	

	Dinner	Snacks	Nutrition
	Empanada-Inspired Salad (page 151) + Rainbow Veggie Pilaf (page 214) + Chimichurri	4 ounces (112g) carrot sticks + 2 tablespoons peanut butter ¼ cup (30g) almonds	**Calories:** 1820 **Fat:** 147.2g **Protein:** 70.9g **Total Carbs:** 72.7g **Net Carbs:** 40.7g
	Lupin Spinach Fritters (page 234) + Yogurt Dill Sauce (page 240) **Balsamic Beets & Greens (page 216) (x2)**	No-Bake White Chocolate–Raspberry Bars (x2) 1 cup (100g) celery sticks + 2 tablespoons peanut butter	**Calories:** 1814 **Fat:** 146.6g **Protein:** 69.3g **Total Carbs:** 73.3g **Net Carbs:** 37.7g
	Lupin Spinach Fritters + Yogurt Dill Sauce + Rainbow Veggie Pilaf (x2)	Pumpkin Spice Breakfast Bars (x2) 2 ounces (56g) carrot sticks + 1 tablespoon peanut butter ¼ cup (30g) almonds	**Calories:** 1824 **Fat:** 148.1g **Protein:** 69.9g **Total Carbs:** 79.5g **Net Carbs:** 38.8g
	Korma-Inspired Cauliflower Bake (page 160) + Rainbow Veggie Pilaf	No-Bake White Chocolate–Raspberry Bars (x2) 2 ounces (56g) carrot sticks + 1 tablespoon peanut butter	**Calories:** 1843 **Fat:** 148.2g **Protein:** 70.5g **Total Carbs:** 76.7g **Net Carbs:** 44.1g
	Korma-Inspired Cauliflower Bake + Rainbow Veggie Pilaf	Pumpkin Spice Breakfast Bars (x2) + 1 tablespoon peanut butter ¼ cup (30g) almonds	**Calories:** 1810 **Fat:** 140.4g **Protein:** 75.1g **Total Carbs:** 93.5g **Net Carbs:** 44.3g
	Cumin Spice "Meatballs" (page 178) **Pumpkin Spice Mashed Butternut Squash (page 230)**	**Raspberry Mini Smoothie Bowl (page 114)** **Dark Chocolate Truffles (page 252) (x4)**	**Calories:** 1703 **Fat:** 130g **Protein:** 71.7g **Total Carbs:** 96.7g **Net Carbs:** 45.5g
	Shepherd's Pie (page 158)	Raspberry Mini Smoothie Bowl ½ cup (60g) almonds	**Calories:** 1803 **Fat:** 143.8g **Protein:** 75.1g **Total Carbs:** 83.2g **Net Carbs:** 44.4g

Week 3 Notes

Day 1: Empanada-Inspired Salad is a variation of the Empanada-Inspired Collard Wraps (page 150). Use leftover plant-based ground and Chimichurri from Week 1.

Day 2: I used So Delicious brand yogurt here. It's a little higher in carbs than CoYo, but it's also less expensive, so it is what I eat when I have more carbs to work with (like in this plan!). I crumble the bars into the yogurt, and it is delightful.

While the yogurt sauce recipe makes four servings, divide it into three portions for serving with the Spinach Lupin Fritters.

If you followed the first two weeks of the plan, you will have leftover Balsamic Vinaigrette for the Balsamic Beets & Greens.

Day 6: Make the Shakshuka with Lupin "Egg" Cups (page 182).

Cumin Spice "Meatballs" are a variation of the Mushroom "Meatballs" (page 178). Pumpkin Spice Mashed Butternut Squash is a variation of the Ras el Hanout Mashed Butternut Squash (page 230). Raspberry Mini Smoothie Bowls are a variation of the Blackberry Yogurt Smoothie Bowl (page 114).

Save one serving of Shakshuka and half of the Dark Chocolate Truffles for Week 4.

Day 7: Save three servings of Shepherd's Pie for Week 4.

Week 3 Ingredients

Produce:

baby spinach, 1 lightly packed cup (30g)

beets with greens, 1 small bunch (about 9 ounces/255g)

bell pepper, red, 1 small (about 2½ ounces/70g)

broccoli stems, 4 ounces (112g)

butternut squash, 1 cup (200g) cubed

carrots, 12 ounces (340g)

cauliflower florets, 2½ pounds (1.2kg)

celery, 1 bunch

chives, 1 small bunch

collard leaves, 4 large

cucumber, 1 medium (about 8 ounces/225g)

dill, 1 bunch

garlic, 12 cloves (or ¼ cup jarred minced garlic)

grape tomatoes, 8 ounces (225g)

lemons, 1½

mint, 1 small bunch

mixed baby greens, 4 cups (120g)

mushrooms, button or cremini, 8 ounces (225g)

onions, 1½ small (about 2½ ounces/70g each)

parsley, 1 large bunch
radishes, 4 ounces (112g)
scallions, 1 bunch
zucchini, 1 medium (about 7 ounces/200g)

Freezer Items:

chopped spinach, 6 ounces (170g)
raspberries, ⅔ cup (60g)
riced cauliflower, 18 ounces (510g)

Refrigerated Items:

coconut yogurt, unsweetened, 3½ cups
    (840ml)
cream cheese, nondairy or dairy, ½ cup (128g)
dairy-free buttery spread, 2 tablespoons, or
    2 additional tablespoons olive oil
lemon juice, 3 tablespoons
pea milk or other nondairy milk of choice,
    1¾ cups (420ml)
plant-based ground, 1½ (1-pound/454-g)
    packages*
prepared yellow mustard, 1 tablespoon

*If you followed the first two weeks of this
plan, you should have a half package of plant-
based ground left over to use for this week.

Pantry Items:

allulose syrup or other sugar-free syrup,
    ¼ cup (60ml)
cacao butter, ½ cup (112g)
canned pumpkin, ¼ cup plus 2 tablespoons
    (90g)
chickpea flour, 2 tablespoons
coconut milk, canned full-fat, ⅔ cup (160 ml)
diced tomatoes, ½ (14½-ounce/411-g) can
extra-virgin olive oil, ¾ cup plus 1 tablespoon
    (195ml)
freeze-dried raspberries, ½ cup (10g)

liquid stevia, ⅜ teaspoon
lupin flour, ¾ cup (90g)
MCT oil or coconut oil, 1 tablespoon
nutritional yeast, ¼ cup (16g)
psyllium husks, 2½ tablespoons
tomato paste, 1 tablespoon
unsweetened chocolate chips, ¼ cup (60g)
vanilla extract, 1 teaspoon
vanilla protein powder, ¾ cup (90g)
vegetable broth, 1 cup plus 3 tablespoons
    (280ml)

Nuts & Seeds:

almond butter, ½ cup (128g)
almonds, 1¼ cups (150g)
chia seeds, 1 teaspoon
ground flaxseed, 2 tablespoons plus 1 teaspoon
hemp seeds, hulled, 2½ cups (400g)
peanut butter, ½ cup (128g)
pumpkin seeds (pepitas), ¼ cup (30g)
sesame seeds, ½ cup (80g)
sunflower seeds, ½ cup (60g)
tahini, ¼ cup (60ml)

Dried Herbs & Spices:

black pepper
black salt (kala namak) or preferred salt
chili powder
dehydrated onion flakes
dried parsley
dried thyme leaves
garam masala
granulated garlic
ground cinnamon
ground cumin
pumpkin pie spice
salt
smoked paprika
white pepper

Week 4: ~45g Net Carbs Daily (Soy-Free)

	Breakfast	Lunch	
Day 1	Shakshuka	Shepherd's Pie	
Day 2	**Chocolate–Peanut Butter Muffins (page 107) (x2)**	Shepherd's Pie	
Day 3	Chocolate–Peanut Butter Muffins (x3)	Peanutty Veggie Noodle Bowl Sesame-Garlic Kale (x2)	
Day 4	**Raspberry Power Smoothie (page 112)**	**Waldorf Kale Salad (page 132) (x2)**	
Day 5	**Blackberry Yogurt Smoothie Bowl (page 114)**	Pistachio Pesto Flatbread (x2) + 1 tablespoon nutritional yeast	
Day 6	**Falafel Waffle (page 98)** + Pistachio Parsley Pesto	Greek Stuffed Peppers + **Ratatouille (page 226) (x2)**	
Day 7	Falafel Waffle + Pistachio Parsley Pesto	Pistachio Pesto Flatbread (x2) + 1 tablespoon nutritional yeast	

Dinner	Snacks	Nutrition
Cumin Spice "Meatballs" (page 178) **Pumpkin Spice Mashed Butternut Squash (page 230) (x2)**	**Flax Crepes with Avocado & Tomato (page 96)** Dark Chocolate Truffles (x4)	**Calories:** 1804 **Fat:** 137.6g **Protein:** 75.2g **Total Carbs:** 106.9g **Net Carbs:** 45.1g
Peanutty Veggie Noodle Bowl (page 164) **Sesame-Garlic Kale (page 212) (x2)**	Flax Crepes with Avocado & Tomato 1 cup (100g) cucumber slices + Pantry Peanut Sauce ¼ cup (30g) almonds	**Calories:** 1859 **Fat:** 150.6g **Protein:** 74.9g **Total Carbs:** 91.1g **Net Carbs:** 36.2g
Shepherd's Pie	Flax Crepes with Avocado & Tomato 1 cup (100g) cucumber slices + Pantry Peanut Sauce	**Calories:** 1903 **Fat:** 153.9g **Protein:** 75.3g **Total Carbs:** 98g **Net Carbs:** 37.2g
Pistachio Pesto Flatbread (page 140) (x2) + 1 tablespoon nutritional yeast	1 cup (100g) cucumber slices + Pantry Peanut Sauce ½ cup (60g) almonds	**Calories:** 1865 **Fat:** 143.8g **Protein:** 70.7g **Total Carbs:** 99.9g **Net Carbs:** 42.1g
Greek Stuffed Peppers (page 148) (x2) Roasted Lemon-Pepper Asparagus	¼ cup (28g) macadamia nuts	**Calories:** 1879 **Fat:** 144g **Protein:** 76.8g **Total Carbs:** 90.1g **Net Carbs:** 45.8g
Pistachio Pesto Flatbread (x2) + 1 tablespoon nutritional yeast	½ cup (60g) almonds	**Calories:** 1864 **Fat:** 145.4g **Protein:** 71.1g **Total Carbs:** 101.5g **Net Carbs:** 46.4g
Greek Stuffed Peppers + Ratatouille (x2)	½ cup (60g) almonds	**Calories:** 1864 **Fat:** 145.4g **Protein:** 71.1g **Total Carbs:** 101.5g **Net Carbs:** 46.4g

Week 4 Notes

Day 1: Use the leftover Shakshuka, Shepherd's Pie, and Truffles from Week 3.

Cumin Spice "Meatballs" are a variation of the Mushroom "Meatballs" (page 178). Pumpkin Spice Mashed Butternut Squash is a variation of the Ras el Hanout Mashed Butternut Squash (page 230).

Day 2: Chocolate–Peanut Butter Muffins are a variation of the PB&J Muffins (page 106).

Replace the tamari with coconut aminos in the Pantry Peanut Sauce to make it soy-free.

Day 4: Raspberry Power Smoothie is a variation of the Raspberry-Beet Power Smoothie (page 112).

Make a double batch of the Pistachio Pesto Flatbread. Sprinkle the flatbread with 1 tablespoon of nutritional yeast. There will be one leftover serving of Roasted Lemon-Pepper Asparagus for dinner on Day 5. At the end of the week, you will have two extra servings of Pistachio Parsley Pesto.

Day 5: Make the Greek Stuffed Peppers using a plant-based ground like Beyond Meat in place of the tempeh, or use a hemp-based, soy-free tempeh.

Week 4 Ingredients

Produce:

asparagus, 1 bunch (about 1 pound/454g)
baby spinach, 1 lightly packed cup (30g)
bell peppers, 1 small, any color (about 2½ ounces/70g) and 2 large red, orange, or yellow (about 6 ounces/170g)
butternut squash, 1 cup (200g) cubed
cauliflower florets, 2 cups (200g)
celery, 1 cup (100g) sliced
cucumber, 1 large (about 10½ ounces/300g)
eggplant, ½ small (about 8 ounces/220g)
garlic, 7 cloves (or 2 tablespoons plus 1 teaspoon jarred minced garlic)

Hass avocado, 1 medium (about 7½ ounces/212g)
jicama, 1 cup (100g) peeled and cubed
kale, 10 cups (210g) chopped
lemon, 1
lime, 1
mushrooms, button or cremini, 8 ounces (225g)
onions, 1½ small (about 2½ ounces/70g)
parsley, 1 large bunch
Roma tomatoes, 3 large (about 3½ ounces/100g each)

scallions, 1 bunch

summer squash or zucchini, 5 medium
(about 7 ounces/200g each)

zucchini noodles, 8 ounces (225g)

Freezer Items:

blackberries, ⅓ cup (50g)

chopped spinach, ⅓ cup (50g)

raspberries, ⅔ cup (60g)

riced cauliflower, 1½ cups (128g)

Refrigerated Items:

chili paste, Sriracha sauce, or hot sauce,
1 teaspoon

coconut yogurt, ½ cup (120ml)

Dijon mustard, 1½ tablespoons

Kalamata olives, 2 ounces (56g)

pea milk or other nondairy milk of choice,
1¾ cups (420ml)

plant-based ground, 8 ounces (225g)

Pantry Items:

apple cider vinegar, 2 tablespoons

baking powder, 1½ teaspoons

baking soda, ¼ teaspoon

coconut aminos, 1 tablespoon

coconut flour, ¼ cup (28g)

coconut oil, 2 tablespoons

extra-virgin olive oil, 1¼ cups plus
2 teaspoons (310ml)

granulated sweetener, 2 tablespoons

liquid stevia, ¼ teaspoon

lupin flour, ¼ cup (60g)

MCT oil or coconut oil, 1 tablespoon

nutritional yeast, 1¾ cups (112g)

psyllium husks, ¼ cup plus 2½ tablespoons
(32g)

toasted sesame oil, 2 tablespoons

tomato sauce, low-sugar, 1 cup (240ml)

unsweetened chocolate chips, 2 tablespoons

vanilla extract, 1 teaspoon

vanilla protein powder, ¼ cup (30g)

vegetable broth, ⅔ cup (160ml)

Nuts & Seeds:

almond butter, ¼ cup (64g)

almonds, 1¾ cups (210g)

chia seeds, 1 teaspoon

ground flaxseed, 1 cup plus 2 tablespoons
plus 1 teaspoon (130g)

hulled hemp seeds, ¼ cup plus 2 tablespoons
plus 1 teaspoon (63g)

macadamia nuts, ¼ cup (28g)

peanut butter, unsweetened, ¾ cup plus
2 tablespoons (224g)

peanuts, ½ cup (60g)

pistachios, raw shelled, ½ cup (60g)

sesame seeds, 1 tablespoon

tahini, ½ cup plus 2 tablespoons (150ml)

walnuts, raw, ½ cup (60g)

Dried Herbs & Spices:

black pepper

dehydrated onion flakes

dried parsley

ginger powder

granulated garlic

Greek seasoning (page 148, or store-bought)

ground cinnamon

ground cumin

herbes de Provence

pumpkin pie spice

red pepper flakes

salt

smoked paprika

References

1. A. Golay, C. Eigenheer, Y. Morel, P. Kujawski, T. Lehmann, T., and N. de Tonnac, "Weight-loss with low or high carbohydrate diet?" *International Journal of Obesity and Related Metabolic Disorders: Journal of the International Association for the Study of Obesity* 20, no. 12 (1996): 1067–72; M. J. Sharman and J. S. Volek, "Weight loss leads to reductions in inflammatory biomarkers after a very-low-carbohydrate diet and a low-fat diet in overweight men," *Clinical Science* (London) 107, no. 4 (2004): 365–9, https://doi.org/10.1042/CS20040111.

2. M. J. Sharman and J. S. Volek, "Weight loss leads to reductions in inflammatory biomarkers after a very-low-carbohydrate diet and a low-fat diet in overweight men," *Clinical Science* (London) 107, no. 4 (2004): 365–9, https://doi.org/10.1042/CS20040111.

3. L. Gupta, D. Khandelwal, S. Kalra, P. Gupta, D. Dutta, and S. Aggarwal, "Ketogenic diet in endocrine disorders: current perspectives," *Journal of Postgraduate Medicine* 63, no. 4 (2017): 242–51, https://doi.org/10.4103/jpgm.JPGM_16_17.

4. E. Brietzke, R. B. Mansur, M. Subramaniapillai, V. Balanzá-Martínez, M. Vinberg, A. González-Pinto, J. D. Rosenblat, R. Ho, and R. S. McIntyre, "Ketogenic diet as a metabolic therapy for mood disorders: evidence and developments," *Neuroscience and Biobehavioral Reviews* 94 (2018): 11–16, https://doi.org/10.1016/j.neubiorev.2018.07.020.

5. V. M. Gershuni, S. L. Yan, and V. Medici, "Nutritional ketosis for weight management and reversal of metabolic syndrome," *Current Nutrition Reports* 7, no. 3 (2018): 97–106, https://doi.org/10.1007/s13668-018-0235-0.

6. M. A. Alzoghaibi, S. R. Pandi-Perumal, M. M. Sharif, and A. S. BaHammam, "Diurnal intermittent fasting during Ramadan: the effects on leptin and ghrelin levels," *PLOS One* 9, no. 3 (2014): e92214, https://doi.org/10.1371/journal.pone.0092214.

7. M. Dirlewanger, V. di Vetta, E. Guenat, P. Battilana, G. Seematter, P. Schneiter, E. Jéquier, and L. Tappy, "Effects of short-term carbohydrate or fat overfeeding on energy expenditure and plasma leptin concentrations in healthy female subjects," *International Journal of Obesity and Related Metabolic Disorders: Journal of the International Association for the Study of Obesity* 24, no. 11 (2000): 1413–8, https://doi.org/10.1038/sj.ijo.0801395.

8. A. Zajac, S. Poprzecki, A. Maszczyk, M. Czuba, M. Michalczyk, and G. Zydek, "The effects of a ketogenic diet on exercise metabolism and physical performance in off-road cyclists," *Nutrients* 6, no. 7 (2014): 2493–508, https://doi.org/ 10.3390/nu6072493.

9. T. Hu, L. Yao, K. Reynolds, T. Niu, S. Li, P. Whelton, J. He, and L. Bazzano, "The effects of a low-carbohydrate diet on appetite: a randomized controlled trial," *Nutrition, Metabolism, and Cardiovascular Diseases*: NMCD 26, no. 6 (2016): 476–88, https://doi.org/10.1016/j.numecd.2015.11.011.

10. T. Hu, K. T. Mills, L. Yao, K. Demanelis, M. Eloustaz, W. S. Yancy, Jr, T. N. Kelly, J. He, and L. A. Bazzano, "Effects of low-carbohydrate diets versus low-fat diets on metabolic risk factors: a meta-analysis of randomized controlled clinical trials," *American Journal of Epidemiology* 176, Suppl 7 (2012): S44–54, https://doi.org/10.1093/aje/kws264.

11. J. Wylie-Rosett, K. Aebersold, B. Conlon, C. R. Isasi, and N. W. Ostrovsky, "Health effects of low-carbohydrate diets: where should new research go?" *Current Diabetes Reports* 13, no. 2 (2013): 271–8, https://doi.org/10.1007/s11892-012-0357-5.

12. University of California - San Francisco, "We know we're full because a stretched intestine tells us so," *ScienceDaily*, accessed February 22, 2021, www.sciencedaily.com/releases/2019/11/191114115918.htm.

13. J. Maljaars, E. A. Romeyn, E. Haddeman, H. P. F. Peters, and A. A. M. Masclee, "Effect of fat saturation on satiety, hormone release, and food intake," *American Journal of Clinical Nutrition* 89, no. 4 (2009): 1019–24, https://doi.org/10.3945/ajcn.2008.27335.

14. C. E. Cherpak, "Mindful eating: a review of how the stress-digestion-mindfulness triad may modulate and improve gastrointestinal and digestive function," *Integrative Medicine* (Encinitas, Calif.) 18, no. 4 (2019): 48–53.

15. H. Ueda, Y. Kikuta, and K. Matsuda, "Plant communication: mediated by individual or blended VOCs?" *Plant Signaling & Behavior* 7, no. 2 (2012): 222–6, https://doi.org/10.4161/psb.18765.

16. D. Aune, E. Giovannucci, P. Boffetta, L. T. Fadnes, N. Keum, T. Norat, D. C. Greenwood, E. Riboli, L. J. Vatten, and S. Tonstad, "Fruit and vegetable intake and the risk of cardiovascular disease, total cancer and all-cause mortality—a systematic review and dose-response meta-analysis of prospective studies," *International Journal of Epidemiology* 46, no. 3 (2017): 1029–56, https://doi.org/10.1093/ije/dyw319.

17. Ibid.

18. M. Imran, F. Ghorat, I. Ul-Haq, H. Ur-Rehman, F. Aslam, M. Heydari, M. A. Shariati, E. Okuskhanova, Z. Yessimbekov, M. Thiruvengadam, M. H. Hashempur, and M. Rebezov, "Lycopene as a natural antioxidant used to prevent human health disorders," *Antioxidants* (Basel, Switzerland) 9, no. 8 (2020): 706, https://doi.org/10.3390/antiox9080706.

19. K. M. Crowe-White, T. A. Phillips, and A. C. Ellis, "Lycopene and cognitive function," *Journal of Nutritional Science* 8 (2019): e20, https://doi.org/10.1017/jns.2019.16.

20. K. E. Senkus, L. Tan, and K. M. Crowe-White, "Lycopene and metabolic syndrome: a systematic review of the literature," *Advances in Nutrition* (Bethesda, Md.) 10, no. 1 (2019): 19–29, https://doi.org/10.1093/advances/nmy069.

21. H. E. Khoo, A. Azlan, S. T. Tang, and S. M. Lim, "Anthocyanidins and anthocyanins: colored pigments as food, pharmaceutical ingredients, and the potential health benefits," *Food & Nutrition Research* 61, no. 1 (2017): 1361779, https://doi.org/10.1080/16546628.2017.1361779.

22. B. W. Lin, C. C. Gong, H. F. Song, and Y. Y. Cui, "Effects of anthocyanins on the prevention and treatment of cancer," *British Journal of Pharmacology* 174, no. 11 (2017): 1226–43, https://doi.org/10.1111/bph.13627.

23. M. G. Choung, I. Y. Baek, S. T. Kang, W. Y. Han, D. C. Shin, H. P. Moon, and K. H. Kang, "Isolation and determination of anthocyanins in seed coats of black soybean (*Glycine max (L.) Merr.*)," *Journal of Agricultural and Food Chemistry* 49, no. 12 (2001): 5848–51, https://doi.org/10.1021/jf010550w.

24. E. Madadi, S. Mazloum-Ravasan, J. S. Yu, J. W. Ha, H. Hamishehkar, and K. H. Kim, "Therapeutic application of betalains: a review," *Plants* (Basel, Switzerland) 9, no. 9 (2020): 1219, https://doi.org/10.3390/plants9091219.

25. B. J. Burri, "Beta-cryptoxanthin as a source of vitamin A," *Journal of the Science of Food and Agriculture* 95, no. 9 (2015): 1786–94, https://doi.org/10.1002/jsfa.6942.

26. B. J. Burri, M. R. La Frano, and C. Zhu, "Absorption, metabolism, and functions of ß-cryptoxanthin," *Nutrition Reviews* 74, no. 2 (2016): 69–82, https://doi.org/10.1093/nutrit/nuv064.

27. E. Aziz, R. Batool, W. Akhtar, S. Rehman, T. Shahzad, A. Malik, M. A. Shariati, A. Laishevtcev, S. Plygun, M. Heydari, A. Rauf, and S. Ahmed Arif, "Xanthophyll: health benefits and therapeutic insights," *Life Sciences* 240 (2020): 117104, https://doi.org/10.1016/j.lfs.2019.117104.

28. K. S. Cho, M. Shin, S. Kim, and S. B. Lee, "Recent advances in studies on the therapeutic potential of dietary carotenoids in neurodegenerative diseases," *Oxidative Medicine and Cellular Longevity* 2018: 4120458, https://doi.org/10.1155/2018/4120458.

29. L. H. Li, J. C. Lee, H. H. Leung, W. C. Lam, Z. Fu, and A. Lo, "Lutein supplementation for eye diseases," *Nutrients* 12, no. 6 (2020): 1721, https://doi.org/10.3390/nu12061721.

30. E. J. Johnson, "Role of lutein and zeaxanthin in visual and cognitive function throughout the lifespan," *Nutrition Reviews* 72, no. 9 (2014): 605–12, https://doi.org/10.1111/nure.12133.

31. G. Wu, Y. Yan, Y. Zhou, Y. Duan, S. Zeng, X. Wang, W. Lin, C. Ou, J. Zhou, and Z. Xu, "Sulforaphane: expected to become a novel antitumor compound," *Oncology Research* 28, no. 4 (2020): 439–46, https://doi.org/10.3727/096504020X15828892654385.

32. Y. Yagishita, J. W. Fahey, A. T. Dinkova-Kostova, and T. W. Kensler, "Broccoli or sulforaphane: is it the source or dose that matters?" *Molecules* (Basel, Switzerland) 24, no. 19 (2019): 3593, https://doi.org/10.3390/molecules24193593.

33. J. Borlinghaus, F. Albrecht, M. C. Gruhlke, I. D. Nwachukwu, and A. J. Slusarenko, "Allicin: chemistry and biological properties," *Molecules* (Basel, Switzerland) 19, no. 8 (2014): 12591–618, https://doi.org/10.3390/molecules190812591.

34. Y. Li, J. Yao, C. Han, J. Yang, M. T. Chaudhry, S. Wang, H. Liu, and Y. Yin, "Quercetin, inflammation and immunity," *Nutrients* 8, no. 3 (2016): 167, https://doi.org/10.3390/nu8030167.

35. Y. Marunaka, R. Marunaka, H. Sun, T. Yamamoto, N. Kanamura, T. Inui, and A. Taruno, "Actions of quercetin, a polyphenol, on blood pressure," *Molecules* (Basel, Switzerland) 22, no. 2 (2017): 209, https://doi.org/10.3390/molecules22020209.

36. H. M. Eid and P. S. Haddad, "The antidiabetic potential of quercetin: underlying mechanisms," *Current Medicinal Chemistry* 24, no. 4 (2017): 355–64, https://doi.org/10.2174/0929867323666160909153707.

37. Norwegian University of Science and Technology, "Eight servings of veggies a day is clearly best for the heart," *ScienceDaily*, accessed May 10, 2021, www.sciencedaily.com/releases/2017/02/170223114807.htm.

38. S. H. Lee-Kwan, L. V. Moore, H. M. Blanck, D. M. Harris, and D. Galuska, "Disparities in state-specific adult fruit and vegetable consumption—United States, 2015," *Morbidity and Mortality Weekly Report* 66, no. 45 (2017): 1241–7, http://dx.doi.org/10.15585/mmwr.mm6645a1.

39. B. Burton-Freeman and H. D. Sesso, "Whole food versus supplement: comparing the clinical evidence of tomato intake and lycopene supplementation on cardiovascular risk factors," *Advances in Nutrition* (Bethesda, Md.) 5, no. 5 (2014): 457–85, https://doi.org/10.3945/an.114.005231.

40. A. van der Vliet, "Cigarettes, cancer, and carotenoids: a continuing, unresolved antioxidant paradox," *American Journal of Clinical Nutrition* 72, no. 6 (2000): 1421–3, https://doi.org/10.1093/ajcn/72.6.1421.

41. S. Wachtel-Galor and I. F. F. Benzie, "Herbal medicine: an introduction to its history, usage, regulation, current trends, and research needs," in *Herbal Medicine: Biomolecular and Clinical Aspects*, 2nd Edition, eds. I. F. F. Benzie and S. Wachtel-Galor (Boca Raton, FL: CRC Press/Taylor & Francis, 2011): Chapter 1.

42. A. Yashin, Y. Yashin, X. Xia, and B. Nemzer, "Antioxidant activity of spices and their impact on human health: a review," *Antioxidants* (Basel, Switzerland) 6, no. 3 (2017): 70, https://doi.org/10.3390/antiox6030070.

43. "What are cruciferous vegetables—and why are they so good for you?" Cleveland Clinic, accessed December 9, 2020, https://health.clevelandclinic.org/crunchy-and-cruciferous-youll-love-this-special-family-of-veggies/.

44. S. M. Tortorella, S. G. Royce, P. V. Licciardi, and T. C. Karagiannis, "Dietary sulforaphane in cancer chemoprevention: the role of epigenetic regulation and HDAC inhibition," *Antioxidants & Redox Signaling* 22, no. 16 (2015): 1382–424, https://doi.org/10.1089/ars.2014.6097.

45. "Mushrooms," The Nutrition Source, accessed March 20, 2020, https://www.hsph.harvard.edu/nutritionsource/food-features/mushrooms/.

46. G. Cardwell, J. F. Bornman, A. P. James, and L. J. Black, "A review of mushrooms as a potential source of dietary vitamin D," *Nutrients* 10, no. 10 (2018): 1498, https://doi.org/10.3390/nu10101498.

47. A. Blagodatski, M. Yatsunskaya, V. Mikhailova, V. Tiasto, A. Kagansky, and V. L. Katanaev, "Medicinal mushrooms as an attractive new source of natural compounds for future cancer therapy," *Oncotarget* 9, no. 49 (2018): 29259, https://doi.org/10.18632/oncotarget.25660.

48. S. Skrovankova, D. Sumczynski, J. Mlcek, T. Jurikova, and J. Sochor, "Bioactive compounds and antioxidant activity in different types of berries," *International Journal of Molecular Sciences* 16, no. 10 (2015): 24673–706, https://doi.org/10.3390/ijms161024673.

49. A. Bouzari, D. Holstege, and D. M. Barrett, "Vitamin retention in eight fruits and vegetables: a comparison of refrigerated and frozen storage," *Journal of Agricultural and Food Chemistry* 63, no. 3 (2015): 957–62, https://doi.org/ 10.1021/jf5058793.

50. J. L. Ivy, "Regulation of muscle glycogen repletion, muscle protein synthesis and repair following exercise." *Journal of Sports Science & Medicine* 3, no. 3 (2004): 131–8.

Allergen Index

 Coconut-free   Nut-free   Peanut-free   Soy-free

Recipes	page	Coconut-free	Nut-free	Peanut-free	Soy-free
Flax Crepes with Avocado & Tomato	96	✓	✓	✓	✓
Falafel Waffles	98	✓	✓	✓	✓
Cabbage & Kale Hash	100	✓	✓	✓	✓
Shakshuka	102	✓	✓	✓	✓
Overnight "N'Oats"	104		✓	✓	✓
PB&J Muffins	106		✓		✓
Pizza Muffins	108		✓	✓	✓
Pumpkin Spice Breakfast Bars	110	✓	✓	✓	✓
Raspberry-Beet Power Smoothie	112	✓	✓	✓	✓
Blackberry Yogurt Smoothie Bowl	114		✓	✓	✓
Garam Masala Spinach Soup	118	✓	✓	✓	✓
Butternut Squash Soup	120		✓	✓	✓
Sauerkraut Soup	122	✓	✓	✓	✓
Fauxtato Leek Soup	124		✓	✓	✓
Cream of Mushroom Soup	126		✓	✓	✓
Shaved Asparagus Salad	128			✓	
Avocado & Grapefruit Kale Salad	130	✓	✓	✓	✓
Waldorf Kale Salad	132	✓		✓	✓
Hemp Seed Tabbouleh	134	✓	✓	✓	✓
Beet Salad with Walnut Dressing	136	✓		✓	✓
Veggie Flatbreads	140	✓	✓	✓	✓
Moroccan-Inspired Butternut Squash Stew	142	✓		✓	✓
Thai-Inspired Cauliflower Coconut Curry	144		✓	✓	
Mushroom Stroganoff	146		✓	✓	✓
Greek Stuffed Peppers	148	✓	✓	✓	
Empanada-Inspired Collard Wraps	150	✓	✓	✓	✓
Cabbage Noodle Chow Mein	152	✓	✓	✓	
Lemony Noodles with Peas & Edamame	154	✓	✓	✓	
Pan-Fried Gnocchi with Garlicky Kale	156		✓	✓	
Shepherd's Pie	158	✓	✓	✓	✓
Korma-Inspired Cauliflower Bake	160		✓	✓	✓
Green Goddess Bowls	162	✓	✓	✓	
Peanutty Veggie Noodle Bowls	164	✓	✓		
Balsamic Roasted Veggie Bowls	166	✓	✓	✓	
Broccoli Noodle Bowls with Peanut Sauce	168	✓	✓		
Basic Baked Tofu	170	✓	✓	✓	
Super Crispy Baked Tofu	172	✓	✓	✓	

Recipes	page				
Tempeh Bacon	174	✓	✓	✓	
Balsamic-Marinated Skillet Tempeh	176	✓	✓	✓	
Mushroom "Meatballs"	178	✓	✓	✓	✓
Vegan Feta	180		✓	✓	
Lupin "Egg" Cups	182	✓	✓	✓	✓
Super Savory Instant Pot Pulled Pork Shoulder	184	✓	✓	✓	
Grilled Chicken Mole	186	✓		✓	✓
Keto Meatballs with Pine Nuts	190	✓		✓	✓
Grilled Marinated Shrimp	192	✓	✓	✓	✓
Crispy Roast Chicken	194	✓	✓	✓	✓
Marinated Pan-Fried Rib Eye	196	✓	✓	✓	✓
Succulent Flank Steak	198	✓	✓	✓	✓
Oven-Roasted New York Strip Steak	200	✓	✓	✓	✓
Sea Vegetable Salad	204	✓	✓	✓	
Green Goddess Broccoli Slaw	206	✓	✓	✓	✓
Greek-Inspired Cucumber Boats	208		✓	✓	
Raw Muhammara	210	✓		✓	✓
Sesame-Garlic Kale	212	✓		✓	✓
Rainbow Veggie Pilaf	214	✓		✓	✓
Balsamic Beets & Greens	216	✓	✓	✓	✓
Harissa Roasted Carrots	218	✓		✓	✓
Roasted Lemon-Pepper Asparagus	220	✓	✓	✓	✓
Chimichurri Roasted Celeriac	222	✓	✓	✓	✓
Pistachio Pesto Brussels Sprouts	224	✓		✓	✓
Ratatouille	226	✓	✓	✓	✓
Broccoli Tots	228	✓	✓	✓	✓
Ras el Hanout Mashed Butternut Squash	230	✓	✓	✓	✓
Tofu Fries	232	✓	✓	✓	
Lupin Spinach Fritters	234	✓	✓	✓	
Taco Fat Bombs	236	✓		✓	✓
Yogurt Dill Sauce	240		✓	✓	✓
Green Goddess Dressing	241	✓	✓	✓	✓
Chimichurri	242	✓	✓	✓	
Pantry Peanut Sauce	243	✓			
Balsamic Vinaigrette	244	✓	✓	✓	✓
Sun-Dried Tomato Dressing	245	✓	✓	✓	✓
Pistachio Parsley Pesto	246	✓		✓	✓
Walnut Dressing	247	✓		✓	✓
Coconut Fakon Bits	248		✓	✓	
Dark Chocolate Truffles	252	✓		✓	✓
Frozen Strawberry Yogurt Bark	254		✓	✓	✓
No-Bake Carrot Cake Bars	256			✓	✓
No-Bake White Chocolate–Raspberry Bars	258	✓		✓	✓
Coconut Matcha Cupcakes	260		✓	✓	✓
Coconut Lime Mousse	262		✓	✓	✓
Cardamom Cauliflower Rice Pudding	264		✓	✓	✓

Recipe Index

Breakfasts

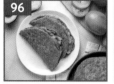
96

Flax Crepes with Avocado & Tomato

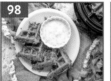
98

Falafel Waffles

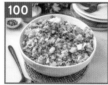
100

Cabbage & Kale Hash

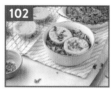
102

Shakshuka

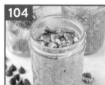
104

Overnight "N'Oats"

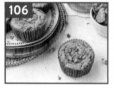
106

PB&J Muffins

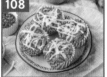
108

Pizza Muffins

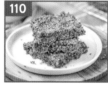
110

Pumpkin Spice Breakfast Bars

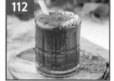
112

Raspberry-Beet Power Smoothie

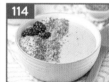
114

Blackberry Yogurt Smoothie Bowl

Soups & Salads

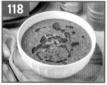
118

Garam Masala Spinach Soup

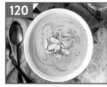
120

Butternut Squash Soup

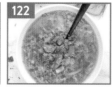
122

Sauerkraut Soup

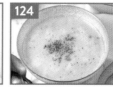
124

Fauxtato Leek Soup

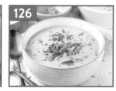
126

Cream of Mushroom Soup

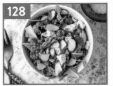 128
Shaved Asparagus Salad

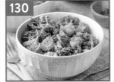 130
Avocado & Grapefruit Kale Salad

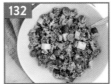 132
Waldorf Kale Salad

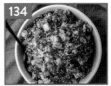 134
Hemp Seed Tabbouleh

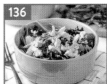 136
Beet Salad with Walnut Dressing

Entrées & Proteins

Entrées

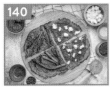 140
Veggie Flatbreads

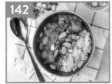 142
Moroccan-Inspired Butternut Squash Stew

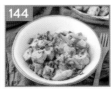 144
Thai-Inspired Cauliflower Coconut Curry

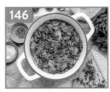 146
Mushroom Stroganoff

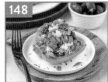 148
Greek Stuffed Peppers

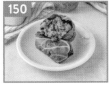 150
Empanada-Inspired Collard Wraps

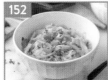 152
Cabbage Noodle Chow Mein

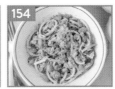 154
Lemony Noodles with Peas & Edamame

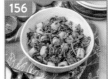 156
Pan-Fried Gnocchi with Garlicky Kale

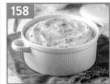 158
Shepherd's Pie

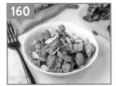 160
Korma-Inspired Cauliflower Bake

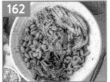 162
Green Goddess Bowls

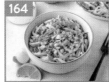 164
Peanutty Veggie Noodle Bowls

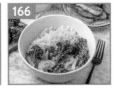 166
Balsamic Roasted Veggie Bowls

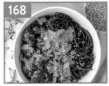 168
Broccoli Noodle Bowls with Peanut Sauce

Protein Toppers

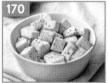
Basic Baked Tofu

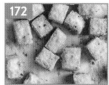
Super Crispy Baked Tofu

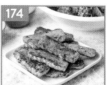
Tempeh Bacon

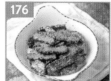
Balsamic-Marinated Skillet Tempeh

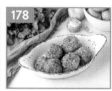
Mushroom "Meatballs"

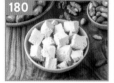
Vegan Feta

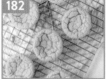
Lupin "Egg" Cups

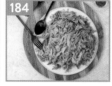
Super Savory Instant Pot Pulled Pork Shoulder

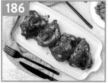
Grilled Chicken Mole

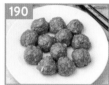
Keto Meatballs with Pine Nuts

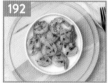
Grilled Marinated Shrimp

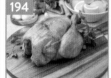
Crispy Roast Chicken

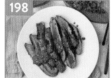
Marinated Pan-Fried Rib Eye

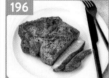
Succulent Flank Steak

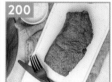
Oven-Roasted New York Strip Steak

Side Dishes & Small Bites

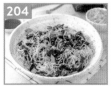

204

Sea Vegetable Salad

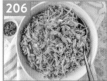

206

Green Goddess
Broccoli Slaw

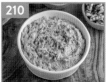

208

Greek-Inspired
Cucumber Boats

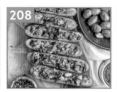

210

Raw Muhammara

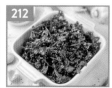

212

Sesame-Garlic Kale

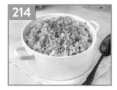

214

Rainbow Veggie Pilaf

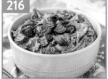

216

Balsamic Beets &
Greens

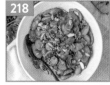

218

Harissa Roasted
Carrots

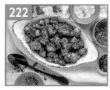

220

Roasted Lemon-
Pepper Asparagus

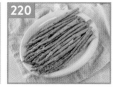

222

Chimichurri Roasted
Celeriac

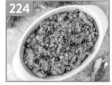

224

Pistachio Pesto
Brussels Sprouts

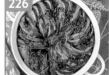

226

Ratatouille

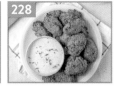

228

Broccoli Tots

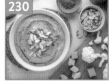

230

Ras el Hanout Mashed
Butternut Squash

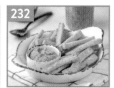

232

Tofu Fries

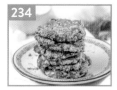

234

Lupin Spinach Fritters

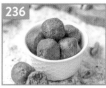

236

Taco Fat Bombs

Sauces & Condiments

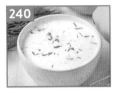
240
Yogurt Dill Sauce

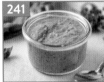
241
Green Goddess Dressing

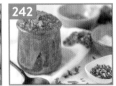
242
Chimichurri

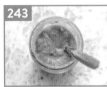
243
Pantry Peanut Sauce

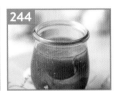
244
Balsamic Vinaigrette

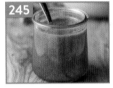
245
Sun-Dried Tomato Dressing

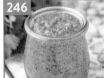
246
Pistachio Parsley Pesto

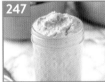
247
Walnut Dressing

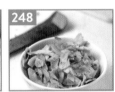
248
Coconut Fakon Bits

Desserts

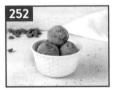
252
Dark Chocolate Truffles

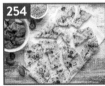
254
Frozen Strawberry Yogurt Bark

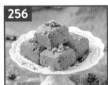
256
No-Bake Carrot Cake Bars

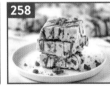
258
No-Bake White Chocolate–Raspberry Bars

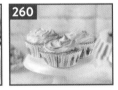
260
Coconut Matcha Cupcakes

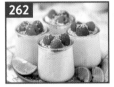
262
Coconut Lime Mousse

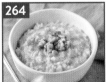
264
Cardamom Cauliflower Rice Pudding

General Index